May the reader have the centered
vision for a great hospital !
Robert Lawrence

*From the dawn of one century*
*to the promise of the next . . .*

# Our Story

## CHARLTON HEALTH SYSTEM

David M. Eskes
writer

Co-Editors:
Earle P. Charlton, II
Frederic C. Dreyer, Jr., LFACHE
Rev. Dr. Robert P. Lawrence

From the dawn of one century to the promise of the next…
Our Story
Charlton Health System

David M. Eskes
writer

Co-Editors:
Earle P. Charlton, II, BA, DBA (Hon.)
Frederic C. Dreyer, Jr., AS, BS, MBA, DBA (Hon.), LFACHE
Robert P. Lawrence, BS,  M. Div., D. Min.

Published by
Heritage Publishers, Inc.
1536 East Maryland Avenue
Phoenix, Arizona 85014-1448
(602) 277-4780

Graphic Design and Production by
inSync Graphic Studio, Inc.
7204 North 16th Street
Phoenix, Arizona 85020-5248
(602) 861-1949

ISBN 0-929690-37-0
Library of Congress Cataloging Number 97-73832

Printed and bound in the United States of America

# Dedication

This book is dedicated to: the families; the people of greater Fall River; trustees; physicians; employees; auxiliary members; volunteers; and all who have cared about this institution and made it possible for the evolving hospital systems to carry out their missions of serving others for one hundred years.

# Contents

# Foreword

*H*ospitals arose in the Middle Ages as institutions for the care and comfort of a heterogeneous population, communities of the poor, insane, frail and maimed, primarily those who lacked family or other social support. "Therapy" was not in the lexicon of those early hospitals; indeed, effective therapy for disease was nonexistent, and the concept of disease itself was vague. Nevertheless, those early hospitals established the highly valued caring function of medicine that we continue to honor today.

American hospitals, of course, did not originate in medieval times but, rather, arose in the late eighteenth and nineteenth centuries. Like their ancient European predecessors, they were caring communities that housed a motley population. The major quality that all of the residents of these early hospitals shared—the lame, blind, mad, dispossessed, and socially dislocated—was poverty. The more privileged and the wealthy suffered at home, cared for by privately employed attendants. Hospitals were viewed as human warehouses, way stations to the grave.

In the middle and late nineteenth century, two great discoveries changed the very nature of medicine and spurred the development of hospitals as centers for the diagnosis and treatment of disease. First, William Morton, in 1846 at the Massachusetts General Hospital, demonstrated the efficacy of ether anesthesia in performing painless major surgery. Although

this accelerated the development of many surgical procedures, post operative infections were so rampant and deadly that surgery remained an often desperate last choice in the physician's therapeutic armamentarium. The reasons for this are obvious to us today as we view pictures of surgeons operating with bare hands and in street clothes, fresh from dismounting from the horse-drawn carriages that had brought them to the hospital.

It was not until the last half of the nineteenth century that growing interest in the "small animals" visible microscopically in putrefying wounds and diseased tissues culminated in the demonstration by Robert Koch in Germany of the "germ" origin of disease and the concept of contagious transmission. Koch identified the bacterium responsible for tuberculosis in 1882 and formulated his four postulates, which remain the foundation of bacteriology to this day. Aseptic and antiseptic surgery soon followed, and the way was opened for the development of antibacterial compounds for the cure of infectious disease, culminating in our modern era of antibiotics.

With the advent of anesthesia and asepsis, hospitals were transformed. Medical research established the causes and natural course of many diseases; therapy became focused and scientific. Also, by the late nineteenth century, the industrial revolution was in full bloom. Massive migration from the

countryside to cities produced large, concentrated populations and enhanced opportunities for the transmission of disease and the creation of epidemics. Family connections were fragmented by the new mobility of populations. Hospitals were required to apply the principles of the new scientific medicine, to isolate contagious individuals, and, often, to replace family support.

The citizens of Fall River responded to these universal trends. Prior to the scientific revolution of the middle and late nineteenth century (in 1835), a "poor farm" was established on the bank of the Taunton River, where the indigent, aged, insane, infirm, and sick languished side by side. In 1885, as a response to the needs of the new medical science, the Fall River Hospital was established for tuberculosis patients; and in 1895 the Fall River Emergency Hospital opened. Consolidation of several of these entities with the Home Training School for Nurses led to the formation of the Union Hospital in 1900, a center for the practice of "modern" medicine in Fall River.

Physicians educated in the new scientific medicine began to emerge from medical schools at the turn of the century. Among these was Philemon Truesdale, an 1898 graduate of the Harvard Medical School and a brilliant surgeon, who began his surgical practice at the City Hospital but soon became disenchanted with the inadequacies of that facility and established his own hospital in a converted rooming house. Dedicated to the practice of the highest quality of modern medicine, Truesdale's enterprise was to grow in size and reputation. Ultimately in 1975, the Truesdale Hospital and its cadre of academically educated specialists would merge with the Union Hospital to form the Charlton Memorial Hospital, a facility embodying the essence of the scientific and technologic development of medicine.

The development and emergence of medicine as we now know it, spans only the last hundred of the thousands of years of human history. We have undoubtedly seen only the beginning of progress that will transform the length of human life, its quality, and its measure of comfort and contentment.

We are justifiably proud of our accomplishments, both locally and globally, but concerns remain and, indeed, have grown in recent years:

Have we failed to extend the benefits of modern medicine to large segments of our communities, particularly the poor and the "uninsured?" Have we neglected the moral obligation to assure the

highest quality of care to all members of society? Are we losing the sense of and commitment to community that characterized the founders of our hospitals?

Have we crossed moral and ethical boundaries in the application of technology? In genetic manipulation? In reproductive innovation? In the management of dying?

Will mega mergers, managed care, for-profit medicine, professional self-interest, and greed associated with great wealth corrupt the practice of medicine and pervert the mission of hospitals?

Contemporary concerns such as these are the product of our successes. Will "success" be our undoing?

Hospitals originated in the Middle Ages as altruistic communities of religious origin. Commitment to civic as well as religious community remained the primary motivation of hospital sponsors into the twentieth century. The founders of the Union Hospital—John D. Flint, Frank S. Stevens, John S. Brayton, and others—were privileged businessmen concerned with the

welfare of the total Fall River population. The generous philanthropy of Earle P. Charlton, combined with the talent of Philemon E. Truesdale, produced another such dedicated institution, the Truesdale Hospital. The challenge ahead is to maintain the traditional humanitarian and communitarian focus of hospitals in an era of rapid expansion, commercialization, and regional and global orientation.

Despite our remarkable scientific advances, care rather than cure is still what we can offer most of our patients. Care is what made medicine a highly valued and esteemed profession for centuries prior to the scientific era. Concern for community built our hospitals. It must remain our focus as we move into a challenging and complex future. ■

—David S. Greer, M.D.
*Dr. Greer was a practicing physician in service to the people of greater Fall River for many years. He is a Nobel Peace Prize winner, past Dean of Brown University School of Medicine, and is currently medical director of Stanley Street Dependency Clinic.*

# Acknowledgements

*A* heartfelt "thank you" is in order to all of those who contributed time, effort, and interviews toward the completion of this project. Particular thanks go to Frederic C. "Rick" Dreyer, who exceeded the call of duty in providing information and materials, often against deadline. Thanks also to the Rev. Dr. Robert P. Lawrence and E.P. "Chuck" Charlton II, whose valuable advice and counsel smoothed out more than one wrinkle. In addition, a debt of gratitude is owed the staffs of the Fall River Historical Society and the Fall River Public Library. Their ready cooperation gave substance to history. Finally, a grateful nod is in order to the late Ernest M. Fell, M.D., whose uncompleted manuscript, "A Short History of the Union Hospital in Fall River," provided a crucial thread of continuity.

The advisory committee assisted the editors in reviewing the drafts of *Our Story* for omissions, deletions, accuracy of names, places, dates and other material within the text and cutlines—a process that seemed endless. With their help we are pleased that the ending goal, publishing the history of Charlton, has been achieved.

## Advisory Committee:

Elizabeth Atwood Lawrence, V.M.D., Ph.D.

Elaine Wilcox, R.N.

Ronald B. Goodspeed, M.D.

Carol A. O'Connell

Edward Boyer

Lillian A. Ferreira

William A. Neilan

Sumner James Waring, Jr.

Anthony Waring

George Bounakis, M.D.

William J.Torpey

Arthur O. Anctil, M.D.

Robert S. Murray

George R. Boyce

David S. Greer, M.D.

Donald H. Ramsbottom

Harvey S. Reback, M.D.

Florence Brigham

Albert L. Michaud

Debra Curless

Mary Ann Wordell, R.N.

Rita N. Wood

John F. Dator

Muriel Mosher

Dorothy A. Allen

Sheila Salvo

Sanford Udis, M.D.

Thomas S. Cinquini

# Preface

There is a oneness about Charlton Health System and its predecessor organizations as described in this historic publication. Throughout its generations, the people associated with Charlton have cared deeply about the institution, one another, and helping others. There have been thousands—volunteers, physicians, and employees—whose individual identities and contributions go far beyond the capacity of this modest publication to document but whose involvement, motivation, and sense of purpose will always be an inseparable part of this outstanding organization. Its hundred-year history is a dramatic story about generations of synchronous, consistent mission and purpose. It is a story that has transcended many generations and organizational models to blend into a whole—a oneness—of humanity and purpose. Regardless of the specific roles or eras they served, or whether the writers at Heritage Publishers and the editors at Charlton were able to identify them individually in this publication, each and every person, from 1894 to 1996, has become an inseparable part of this oneness of time and mission.

From the "cottage industry" of the 1880s to "managed care" 2000, each generation has demonstrated extraordinary resourcefulness and creativity as it has continuously transformed itself into whatever form has been necessary to best carry out its constant purpose and mission. From the early stages, when sick and injured people were treated in renovated old houses, to today's sophisticated hospitals and free-standing health-promotion and medical-service facilities, outreach programs, and large regional systems, Charlton has earned the respect of its patients and the public at large as a compassionate, competent, and quality provider of health and medical education and services. It entered into mergers in 1900, 1975, and 1996 and today is part of Southcoast Health System, serving the greater Fall River–New Bedford–Wareham areas and the region beyond.

As with generations past, those to come will face new transformations in the form of mega mergers and vast expansions of regional, national and international systems. Although the process of anticipating the future will continue and transformations of organizational form and substance will be contemplated and developed, the oneness, which has been Charlton with its mission of caring and serving others, must be preserved and perpetuated. ∎

Frederic C. Dreyer, Jr., LFACHE
President Emeritus and Hon. Trustee
Southcoast Health System

# Beginnings

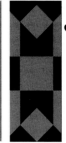

## Chapter One

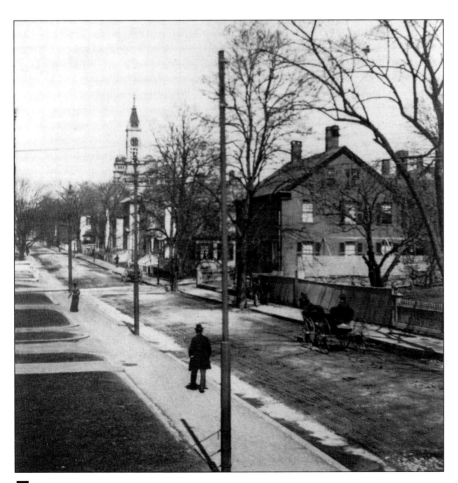

■ *Fall River site where the Emergency Hospital would be built in 1895.*

*R*ose Silvia's scalp was torn off when they brought her into Fall River's Union Hospital that winter day in 1902. The young worker had caught her hair in a spinning shaft at Marshall's Hat Factory and was bleeding profusely. Dr. William A. Dolan labored at first to save her life, then later to repair the damage to her skull with skin grafts donated by local citizens. It provided good copy for the Fall River newspapers, which kept up a running account of her slow recovery as Dolan worked diligently to attach the tiny bits of tissue. Hat factory owners even paid male employees "up to $100 each" for contributing skin.

In a way, Rose Silvia was lucky. If the accident had happened just a decade earlier, she might have died. Medicine had come a long way. By 1902 hospitals were cleaner, physicians more knowledgeable, and surgeons more skillful. The palette of healing arts offered a much wider array of services. Odd as it may seem, the young woman had Fall River industry to thank for her good fortune, as well as her bad. If not for industry leaders such as John D. Flint, Frank S. Stevens, and John S. Brayton, the fully equipped Union Hospital would not have been there to receive her.

When seventy-four-year-old John D. Flint and his fellow community leaders gathered about a table in the home of Elias A. Tuttle on a humid August evening in 1900, they could not have foreseen the ripple effect of what

## John D. Flint

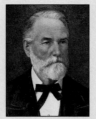

John D. Flint, president, Union Hospital, 1900-1901 1904-1905

When budding entrepreneur John Dexter Flint peddled tin on the rutted streets of Fall River in the 1840s, he is said to have lived an entire week on twenty-three cents. While it is true that Flint could squeeze a nickel, the anecdote belies his generosity as a community leader and philanthropist. By the time he died in 1907 at the age of eighty-one, he had amassed a fortune through retail, banking, textile mills, and land speculation. Were it not for John D. Flint, Union Hospital and a host of other civic undertakings in Fall River might never have seen the light of day. It was Flint who presided over the creation of Fall River Hospital in 1885 and served as its first president. It was Flint who—anticipating the demands of a new century—merged Fall River Hospital with the Emergency Hospital and Home Training School for Nurses in 1900 to create Union Hospital.

Born in 1826 to a humble farm family in Reading, Massachusetts, Flint started his career as a tin peddler at the age of nineteen for Benjamin Cunningham, a Fall River businessman. In those days of laissez faire capitalism, it was not enough for an aspiring lad to work seven days a week, to scrimp and save—everyone did that. Success required heavy doses of ambition and cunning. Flint did not want for either. By the time he was twenty-three, he was a partner in Cunningham's firm. By twenty-eight, he was sole owner. Flint soon took on new partners and expanded the business to include carpeting and furniture. In 1871 he bought two farms in east Fall River totaling sixty-five acres. They later became the site for two textile mills and Flint Village, a tenement district housing thirty thousand workers. As time went on, Flint added to his wealth by investing in several local mills and banks. He served as director or trustee for a number of these enterprises, as well as for the Fall River Railroad. Flint also owned several city blocks teeming with lucrative commercial concerns and tenements.

In many ways, Flint mirrored the rags-to-riches story of other nineteenth century entrepreneurs. He was self-made, staunchly religious (Methodist), shaped by a pious mother, and reform-minded in a moral sense. For example, Flint was a director for the Y.M.C.A., Home for the Aged, Salvation Army, Fall River Boys' Club, and Gospel Rescue Mission. He and his wife, Clarissa, were antislavery activists and lifelong prohibitionists. His investment of time and money in the community stemmed not only from a paternal sense of obligation but enlightened self-interest. In an indirect fashion, his generosity paid personal dividends. Flint, a sufferer of painful stomach disorders, likely had his life extended several years via surgical procedures expedited by his—and others'—support of medicine.

Perhaps Flint's diplomatically crafted obituary in *The Fall River Herald News* said it best: "His was in some respects a peculiar temperament. He was a born trader. To make money was perhaps the first instinct throughout his busy life. As a rule he did not get the worst of a bargain. Success achieved, his next purpose in life seemed to be how to do good with his gains. He was without question the most generous giver in the city."

they were about to do. The task at hand was clear: form a corporation for the consolidation of Fall River Hospital and Emergency Hospital into a new entity, Union Hospital. It was a practical matter for these Victorian gentlemen of stern mien. Yet the impact of that decision still touches Fall River and its environs. It was a far-reaching move that was to influence a century of health care through wars, epidemics, and economic strife. It set the tone for a community health system that would prove uncommonly responsive over the years.

If Flint, a self-made real-estate magnate, was far sighted, he also had the benefit of a strong wind at his back. It was called change. America and Fall River were sailing into the twentieth century, and life would not wait. Flint had felt the first stirrings of those winds fifteen years before, when he spearheaded the drive to create Fall River Hospital. Even then textile mills lined the Taunton River like sentinels, and the city hummed with activity. The Civil War was a recent memory, and the era of expansion was in full swing. The Fall River textile industry, already a thriving concern, began to grow almost exponentially as demand for cotton soared.

Most of the Irish settlers who worked the mills in earlier decades had segued into business and government, a migration in itself. They had been replaced by legions of French-Canadian immigrants and growing pockets of other ethnic groups, notably the Portuguese. Immigration, which had swelled the population of Fall River to more than 56,000, was reweaving the fabric of Fall River society and imposing urban demands on a social structure more attuned to pastoral, midcentury transcendentalism. A newspaper article from that era relates how a fire devastated the public library, an antiquated firetrap packed cheek-by-jowl with 31,000 volumes. The lack of preparedness is telling.

Perhaps the greatest surprise to all will be the announcement that not a cent's worth of insurance was carried upon the building. For many years this city did insure its buildings in part, but the expense was heavy, and for some years insurance of public buildings has been given up and the policies allowed to elapse as they became due.

It was symptomatic of an engrained Yankee frugality that pervaded many aspects of life in Fall River, particularly those of business and labor. The frugality was combined with a paternalistic approach to governing that was as doomed as the antebellum South. The era of fourteen-hour days, subsistence wages, and child labor were numbered, a fact not lost on Fall River's more perceptive leaders. In 1885 events were taking place in other parts of the world that would hasten that denouement. Volume two of Karl Marx's *Das Kapital* was published, George Eastman introduced coated photographic paper, Karl Benz perfected a single-cylinder engine for the "horseless carriage," and France's Louis Pasteur developed a vaccine for rabies. Moreover, the first successful cholecystectomy (the surgical removal of a gall bladder) was performed.

The last accomplishment, though understated, was of considerable significance to industrial Fall River, where health care was a growing issue. It was one of a string of surgical advances during the decade that would ultimately lift the medieval hulks of hospitals into drydock and refit them as flagships of modern medical technology. No longer would they be viewed as warehouses for dying indigents. They would be perceived as sanctuaries of healing—a far cry from the traditional, rat-infested "poor farms" where the indigent, aged, infirm, and sick languished side by side, forgotten. Fall River's first hospital, in fact, is reported to have been on a poor farm established in 1835 on the banks of the Taunton River. In 1851 an official city hospital was erected on the same site, which borders Brownell Street between North Main Street and Highland Avenue.

During the Civil War, the reputation of hospitals surged briefly when Clara Barton, founder of the American Red Cross, and other health officials stressed recovery, humane treatment, and systemized cleanliness in treating the wounded and sick. This was as much for ethical as scientific reasons. At the time, cause and effect were largely determined by on-the-job observation. Practice, rather than scientific inquiry, dictated that latrines be separated from food and water to prevent contamination.

It was not until the latter part of the century, when medical science bloomed, that hospitals began to be accepted by the public as centers of healing. The new Fall River Hospital, located on Prospect Street, was in the vanguard of that transformation. From its inception in 1885, it was well-managed and embraced the entire community. Its corporate and board members represented a relatively broad spectrum of Fall River society. Many, like Flint, came from humble origins. Flint was elected president of the corporation; Stevens, vice president; Charles J. Holmes, treasurer; and Marcus G. B. Swift, clerk. There were eighteen members on the initial board of trustees, including the above officers. A year later, 126 new members were elected to the corporation.

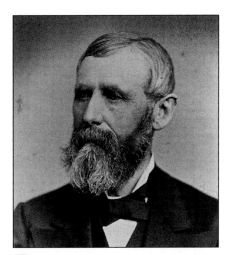

Dr. Robert T. Davis, president, Union Hospital, 1902-1904

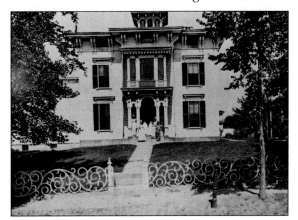

Fall River Hospital

Although Fall River Hospital depended for its support in large part on donations from affluent benefactors, it also sponsored public fund-raisers through excursions, receptions, entertainment, and the like. It offered "free beds," which could be purchased by affluent citizens for $5,000 each. The beds guaranteed "care in perpetuity" for indigents (the first buyer was one Mary Young). In 1888 the trustees created the Woman's Board, a volunteer organization that would play a crucial support role in coming years. Meanwhile, the hospital continued to expand in an effort to meet community needs. It acquired the Valentine estate on 72 Prospect Street in 1887, added a west wing to its hospital residence in 1891, established the Training School for Nurses in 1888, and included a maternity ward in 1891. One unique addition was the Jersey cow "Nellie," which trustee and cattle fancier Frank Stevens thoughtfully donated.

While Fall River Hospital negotiated the shoals of financial solvency and public demand, other Fall River medical facilities began to appear. A new city hospital was opened in 1894, as well as a city clinic and the Contagious Disease Hospital for tubercolus patients. That same year, Dr. John H. Gifford, assisted by Elizabeth H. Brayton, established the Home Training School for Nurses at the corner of Rock and Franklin streets, opposite the present-day Central Congregational Church. The mission of the school, which offered a two-year course, was to provide nurses for homes. It mirrored reality. "There is in our city today," its first annual report read, "ten times as many people sick at home as are sick in hospitals."

In 1895 the Fall River Emergency Hospital opened, with the primary goal of assisting the steadily increasing number of accident victims. Affiliated with the Home Training School for Nurses, it shared the same property in the center of the city. By 1897, however, Emergency Hospital was rendering another service that saved not only lives but precious time as well. As the new bacteriological testing facility for typhoid and diphtheria, it eliminated the need to send specimens all the way to Boston. Despite this and other medical gains over the past decade, social conditions in Fall River indicated that the status quo would not meet demands of the new century looming just over the horizon. Flint anticipated this and began moving toward consolidation.

After the August meeting to incorporate, Flint and his colleagues moved quickly to get Union Hospital started. An organizational meeting was held in September, followed by the chartering on October 1. Flint was elected president of the board of trustees; Robert C. Kerr, vice president; and Richard P. Borden, treasurer. Anticipating future

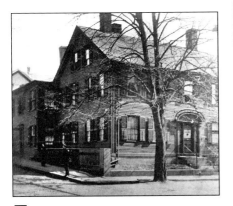

Emergency Hospital, still standing on the corner of Main and Cherry Streets

## John S. Brayton

When conditions permitted, John Summerfield Brayton liked to cross the Taunton River and visit his farm holdings in south Somerset. The bucolic nineteenth century setting provided welcome relief from the bustle of industrial Fall River.

Brayton, who had started his professional life as a lawyer and later acquired a fortune in business, was a contemplative man of many parts: mill owner, historian, banker, farmer, and lawyer. He was deeply conservative and cautious—a man who did not invest in enterprises unless convinced of their viability.

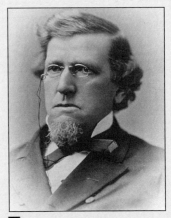

Hon. John S. Brayton, president, Union Hospital, 1901-1902

But when his fellow businessmen, led by John D. Flint, decided to establish the Fall River Hospital, Brayton unhesitatingly signed on as a trustee. And when Fall River Hospital merged with Emergency Hospital to form Union Hospital, Brayton not only served as president (1901-02) but donated an acre of his estate to the institution. By his actions, Brayton helped—along with his contemporaries—to give Union its strong identification as a community hospital.

Brayton was born December 3, 1826, in Swansea of a farm family. After graduating from Brown University in 1851, he studied law at Harvard University. In 1854 he became city solicitor of Fall River and three years later was elected Bristol County clerk. Brayton quit the practice of law in 1868 to assume managership of his sister's estate, a string of industrial enterprises inherited from her late husband, Bradford Durfee. Over the years, his careful stewardship expanded the holdings and placed him among the preeminent leaders of Fall River.

A staunch Congregationalist, Brayton supported churches of several denominations. In his spare time, he pursued his hobby of compiling local history and is said to have known more about Fall River's past than any person alive. Following his death, his son, John S. Brayton II, served as a trustee of Union Hospital. His grandson, John S. Brayton III, served as a trustee and president of the board from 1942 to 1961. ■

expansion, trustee John S. Brayton donated an acre of land to the hospital on the northwest corner of Prospect and Hanover streets. In November 330 members of the former Fall River Hospital and Home Training School for Nurses were unanimously elected as members of the new corporation. In addition, the women's boards were combined.

The new hospital was still housed in the old Flint residence, a vestige of the nineteenth-century cottage-industry tradition. But its staff of twenty-six physicians now offered specialties in "diseases of the eye, ear, skin, nose and throat and genitourinary." There also was a gynecologist on staff plus several surgeons and general physicians. This centralized grouping of specialists was ahead of its time and foreshadowed the comprehensive nature of health care that Union Hospital and its successors would provide the Fall River community. Dr. Lucy C. Hill was the only woman on staff, but over the years, Union Hospital would employ a substantial number of women physicians. The first annual report for the hospital

tallied 372 inpatients. Of 765 outpatients, 463 were from the mills, 141 private, 35 free, and 126 rebate (discount). Bed capacity was thirty. Union was the first nonprofit hospital in the area.

The consolidated nursing program, now called the Union Hospital Training School, counted sixty-one students that first year. Nurses received, in addition to board and room, an allowance of $75 the first year and $100 the second plus three weeks' paid vacation and one week of sick leave. The criteria for being accepted in the program included "good character, a common school education and physical capacity" (read endurance). The hours may have been long and the duties sometimes onerous, but it undoubtedly beat working in the mills.

No sooner had Union Hospital gotten under way than plans emerged for a larger, tailor-made edifice that would accommodate one hundred patients and fifty private rooms. In 1902 the planning committee, composed of Elias A. Tuttle, Dr. Robert T. Davis, and Dr. Richard Thompson, sought expertise by visiting hospitals in New York and Boston. A few months later, a down payment of $1,000 was made to the Boston

architectural firm of Kendall, Taylor, and Stevens. It was estimated the new building would cost $80,000 to $100,000. Thirty-thousand dollars was pledged at the outset.

The increasing demands on medical facilities such as Union Hospital proved hospitals in general had turned the corner. The emergence of anesthesia and antisepsis had set the stage. Now technology was the driver. Surgery had advanced to the point where it had to be done in a specially equipped medical facility. In addition, private rooms were inching up in popularity and becoming excellent sources of revenue. More and more citizens sought treatment in hospitals as a matter of course. The epithet "sawbones" was largely dead. The public had come not only to respect the medical profession but sometimes stand in awe of it. This attitude would not change in Fall River.

# A New Century

By 1900 Fall River had evolved into a textile colossus, employing 26,372 workers and producing 843 million yards of cloth annually. The peak had yet to be reached. The heavy concentration of industry and immigrants—eighteen nations were represented—made Fall River the diversity capital of the nation for a city of its size. In fifteen short years it had doubled its population to more than one hundred thousand. With three million

spindles humming night and day against the backdrop of billowing smokestacks, the moniker "Spindle City" was not an exaggeration. Fall River had great wealth and great expectations—even great soirees.

During the first year of the new century, Fall River hosted the likes of Maud Gonne, Irish feminist and cofounder of Sinn Fein; and Winston Churchill, the youngest member of the House of Commons and a hero of the Boer War. Fortunately, Gonne, who was raising funds for the Boers, visited in February and Churchill in December. "For fifty minutes," a local newspaper reported, "Churchill detailed his experiences in an escape from Pretoria to Delagoa Bay and later his experience as a soldier going back to Pretoria [and presumably, the cavalry charge at Omdurman]. Those who heard him say his manner is as frank as a schoolboy's. It would not be surprising if an effort is made to have him appear here in public later on."

Just down society hill and out of sight, however, lay mind-boggling poverty, disease, and ignorance. A few short years before, an affronted minister had declared, "A photograph would shock the world." Sanitation was almost unheard of in workers' quarters, where raw sewage collected in scraggly yards and ran down the street. Toilets were often stopped up for lack of water. Worst of all, the infant mortality rate exceeded two hundred deaths per thousand births, one of the highest in the nation. As late as 1910, an investigation of ten thousand homes by the Fall River Board of

Health found nearly half of them unfit for habitation. If uneducated parents were guilty of ignorance in disregarding cleanliness, wealthy absentee landlords were plainly derelict for installing crude, unworkable plumbing in an attempt to save money.

The jobsite was not any better. Long hours and exhausting repetition dulled the reflexes and triggered industrial accidents. Workers were routinely maimed, sometimes even killed. Labor committees complained of knee-deep water and air thick with cotton fibers, hair, and sand. Common cups were used to dip drinking water from barrels of stagnant water. In one case, a Fall River doctor testified that the barrel was frequently scrubbed with the same mop used for the "water closets." Topping it off, textile "operatives" were the lowest-paid workers of any industry. For the most part, management did not feel an obligation to improve the situation. This was the Gilded Age, the age of pure capitalism. It was every man for himself. Simeon B. Chase, a respected Fall River manufacturer, put it this way: "I may be old-fashioned, but I am a little Calvinistic in my theories. I think life means something besides trying to make the road easier for everybody."

There were those who did not fully agree with Chase and his contemporaries. They included not only factory workers but people in high places. President Theodore Roosevelt, himself no stranger to wealth, broke up monopolies and championed reform. Steel magnate

## Frank S. Stevens

In 1878 the Fall River textile industry was rocked by a financial scandal that rendered many mill stocks worthless. Community leaders feared the worst—plummeting confidence, followed by total economic collapse. One leader, Frank Stevens, had a different take.

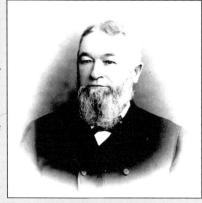

*Frank Shaw Stevens*

"Boys," he said, lighting up a cigar, "I have driven six horses on a stagecoach in California, and I can do it again. You can't break me." Stevens, one of Fall River's wealthiest businessmen, was not posturing. He had made one fortune in the California Gold Rush of 1849 and another during the textile boom of the 1870s. He had tasted life in all its varieties, giving him a broader perspective than most of his Fall River peers.

Stevens immediately assumed treasurership of the Davol and Mechanics mills, personally endorsed their notes, and backed them with his own money. Confidence was soon restored, and the notes were paid—the crisis was over. The fact that some of Stevens' money came from liquor interests elicited not one wagging finger from his temperance-minded Fall River colleagues. Frank Stevens had put his neck on the line for Fall River and ... well, Frank was different.

Frank Shaw Stevens was born in Vermont in 1827 to a stage driver and a mother who died when he was five years old. He was raised by his uncle and aunt, who owned a tavern. Stevens left home at fifteen and eventually headed west to the gold fields, where he teamed up with Providence resident James Birch to start a stagecoach line. California was overrun with gold seekers, and the need for transportation was desperate. In one month, for example, the San Francisco Customs House tallied $29 million in gold. Within a few years, the young entrepreneurs were rich. In 1857 the partnership ended tragically when the colorful Birch drowned off Cape Hatteras on a voyage from San Francisco to New York. Stevens married his widow, Julia, left California, and eventually settled in her home village of Swansea. After Julia died in 1871, Stevens married Elizabeth Case.

Stevens was straight out of a Brett Harte short story. He was a flamboyant man with brains and charm enough to bedazzle polite society—at ease in salon or saloon. He was a lover of horses and a soft touch for anyone down on his luck. The people of Fall River held him in awe. Stevens, along with John D. Flint, Charles Holmes, and Marcus Smith, was a founder of Fall River Hospital (1885) and its first vice president. Later he served as a director. He also served as a state senator. A generous private giver, Stevens had just begun a program of public philanthropy when he died in 1898, leaving Elizabeth to carry it out. In coming years, her support of Union Hospital would prove critical. ■

## Elizabeth R. Stevens

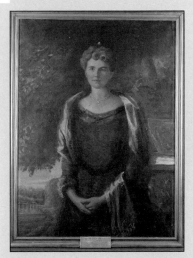

■ *Elizabeth R. Stevens*

Those who knew Elizabeth Stevens remember her as a beautiful, elegantly coiffed woman who wore a tiara and exuded a regal air. She was "brilliant," one observer said. "She looked like all the queens you ever saw."

The role could have come from central casting, and Stevens played it well. She was a woman who knew her place, which was "administrator-in-chief" of the Stevens fortune. She knew her priorities, and Frank Stevens always topped the list. Legend has it, in fact, that she "stole" the millionaire widower from her younger sister, Mary.

Despite being twenty-two years younger than her husband, Elizabeth proved an excellent mate. The couple lived lavishly and provided excellent copy for local society reporters, who kept a running tally of their comings and goings, whether shopping trips to Boston, vacations in Saint Augustine, or excursions on their steam yacht, Julia. Yet the Stevenses had the common touch, counting as friends everyone from U.S. presidents to local mill workers.

Elizabeth Stevens was born in Swansea in 1849. A graduate of the Normal School in Bridgewater, she taught school briefly before marrying in 1873. Although Stevens lived a "red velvet life," she was an energetic woman of diverse interests who was not content to merely measure her life in soirees. After her husband's death, she expanded his fortune six fold, thanks to shrewd real-estate deals and the sage advise of business confidant, Robert S. Goff. She was a staunch friend of Union Hospital, providing much-needed financial support on a regular basis.

At her death in 1930, the Stevens estate was valued at $6 million. The more than sixty bequests to libraries, churches, schools, and social agencies took up an entire page in a local newspaper. Stevens provided for everyone, right down to the servants. Union Hospital's gift totaled some $350,000, while servant Margaret Duncan was guaranteed the income from a $10,000 trust if she continued "in the employ of my said sister." "Said sister" Mary received $1 million plus all real-estate holdings and use of the Stevens estate for life. Nobody ever said Elizabeth Stevens was not fair. ■

Andrew Carnegie urged fellow millionaires, in his article, "Wealth," to administer their money through public trusts while still alive. Down in the trenches, labor unions pushed reform and launched crippling strikes, nowhere more potently than in Fall River itself. "Muckraking" journalists Upton Sinclair, Ida Tarbell, and Lincoln Steffens unmasked corporate abuses with such works as *The Jungle*, A *History of the Standard Oil Company*, and *Shame of the Cities*. Their readers, a growing and influential middle class, demanded change.

In a speech at Fall River's Bijou Theatre in 1904, socialist Eugene Debs declared that "capitalism has ... outlived its usefulness." Debs railed against overproduction and the "three million children employed in the sweatshops, the factories and mines." He even alarmed the rowdy audience by predicting the time would come when women would be able to vote, live independently, and provide for themselves. Debs never had a chance at the election box, but he beamed a light into the future. And establishment figures like former U.S. Attorney General Albert E. Pillsbury picked up on it.

Enlightened industrialists, Pillsbury said at the dedication of the Swansea Public Library in 1900, "will not wait for the rude hand of the law to cut down or scatter their fortunes, but will choose voluntarily to administer their own estates in recognition of the obligations of wealth to the community." Elizabeth R. Stevens, who had funded the library,

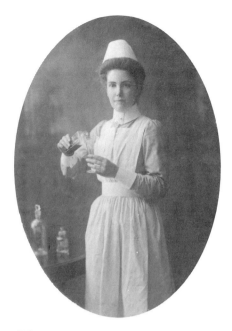

*Nurse Jessie Christie, circa 1910 who eventually worked at Union Hospital in the maternity ward.*

needed no convincing. She and her late husband, Frank, always had been ahead of the curve. Even as she listened to Pillsbury speak, Mrs. Stevens was mapping out a strategy for her philanthropic campaign. Union Hospital was part of it.

Wealthy benefactors may have been abundant in Fall River, but they were not in a position to foot the bill for everything. To sustain philanthropy, wealth must be nurtured and conserved. The leaders at Union Hospital respected this elemental fact. When the fledgling institution nearly ran aground financially during its initial years, Richard P. Borden, a young trustee, incorporated a group of some three hundred citizens to whom the board of trustees would be ultimately responsible. The object was to dispel any suspicions of elitism in regard to the hospital and include

the citizenry in the governing process. The tactic worked. The citizens, given a say in how the hospital would be run, showed its appreciation by pitching in to raise the money necessary to get Union Hospital back on course.

Not everything was resolved so expeditiously in those early years. In 1901 student nurses at Union Hospital rebelled when ordered by the board of trustees to relocate to the Home Training School for Nurses, formerly part of the Emergency Hospital before merger. The nurses viewed their removal to another site as a violation of their contract with the old Fall River Hospital, which assured their place of employment. The result was a stalemate. The obstacle was finally overcome but not before the resentful nurses were evicted from their quarters.

Perhaps, in view of nursing conditions, the nurses' anger should be taken in context. According to The American General Hospital by Elizabeth Long and Janet Golden, student nurses at the turn of the century provided virtually free labor to hospitals. Despite their increasing clinical proficiency, they tended to be stereotyped as skilled domestics by male medical colleagues. They were "helpmates" who made bandages, changed dressings, treated bedsores, administered enemas, gave baths, and applied line splints. Sometimes they even cooked for patients. Through it all, they were expected to be relentlessly cheerful, fulfilling the cultural role assigned to them.

But there were light moments, too—albeit inadvertently—as

shown by this newspaper report from March 27, 1906: "James Holmes, 21 years of age, employed as a weaver at the Davis Mills, is in critical condition at the Union Hospital as a result of swallowing his teeth while at dinner yesterday." The culprit, it seems, was Holmes' upper partial, which unexpectedly dislodged, causing him to swallow it. Dr. B.G. Schofield, assisted by two other doctors, performed "delicate surgery" to remove the offending item and expressed hope that the patient would recover.

House rules at Union Hospital were in some ways stricter, in other ways looser, than modern regulations—a reflection, perhaps, of late Victorian culture. For example, anyone "having acute venereal disease or alcoholism" could not be admitted "except as a paying patient." "Profane or obscene language, objectionable literature, loud talking and incivility" were strictly prohibited on pain of discharge. Yet "tobacco, wine or intoxicating liquors" were allowed by consent of the physician in attendance. In addition, donations to the hospital in those early days could be downright homey, as indicated by a Union annual report listing, among more prosaic items, pickles, jelly, eggs, turnips, an American flag, fruit, and a barrel of flour.

# A Man Named Truesdale

*W*hile Union Hospital was getting its sea legs, a tall, young Fall River surgeon by the name of Philemon Edwards Truesdale quietly purchased the rectory of Sacred Heart Church on the corner of Winter and Pine streets in 1905 for $12,000 from Fr. James E. Cassidy. His object was to establish a private surgical hospital. Dr. Truesdale, an 1898 graduate of Harvard Medical School, had interned at Boston Hospital before coming home to practice—first at City Hospital, then in a converted rooming house and finally, the Davol house on Main Street. As a surgeon, Dr. Truesdale was regarded as brilliant.

Brilliant or not, it was considered a breach of propriety in those days for a doctor to run a surgical hospital. And private hospitals were frowned on. Dr. Truesdale's detractors—there were several—airily dismissed him as knife-happy. In a professional sense, he was. Philemon Truesdale was first, last, and always a surgeon. In fact, it was the lack of surgical opportunity in other Fall River institutions that drove him to start his own hospital. Dr. Truesdale sought only the best doctors for his new enterprise, hiring the highly regarded Dr. John H. Gifford and Dr. William T. Learned as assistants. He also hired six nurses and a secretary-treasurer. With little capital to spare, the enthusiastic young surgeon and his staff hung out their shingle.

Business took off immediately. In a stroke of luck, one of Truesdale's earliest patients was young Perry Charlton, who was rushed to the hospital with a ruptured appendix and peritonitis—an often fatal complication at the time. The Truesdale staff managed to save the boy's life, earning the undying gratitude of his father, Earle P. Charlton, a successful local retail entrepreneur. In coming years, the elder Charlton would impact Fall River's medical establishment in ways that would touch every citizen. He would contribute to a medical saga that spanned seven decades and inspired both excellence and enmity between two major hospitals. Dr. Truesdale could not know it, but the seeds of competition had been planted in the former rectory. There would be no turning back.

# Saint Anne's Debutes

*A* year after Philemon Truesdale opened the doors of his little hospital, Fall River became home to another hospital, Saint Anne's, which was built and paid for by the France-based Dominican Sisters of the Presentation. Located on the southeast corner of South Main and Middle streets, the hospital boasted three stories and 11,824 square feet. It could accommodate up to 125 patients. The cost of the project was $100,000. Then, as now, Saint Anne's served mostly residents of French-Canadian extraction concentrated on the south side of Fall River. "The interior of the hospital," said a 1906 newspaper article, "is ... a wealth of room, light and air." "The private rooms," it added, "will be the largest of any hospital in these parts. The doctors who have visited the operating room say that it is unsurpassed by any."

# Union Gets a New Home

*I*n 1908 Union Hospital finally moved into its new quarters on Prospect and Hanover streets. Called the Main Building (now Borden), the four-story red-brick building with its two-story east and west wings provided the room and facilities needed to meet the demands of a ballooning population. The east wing housed open (free) wards for the poor, while the west wing contained private wards. Main included administration, surgical, recovery, labor, and delivery areas plus an emergency-treatment room and other medical services. Judging by a local newspaper report, the hospital was a modern marvel. "There are seventy-eight beds for patients," the article read.

Beside every one there is a connection for attaching an electric plug to secure a current for electrical treatment, foot warming or any kindred purpose. Every patient's bed is also equipped with a signal wire with which the patient may call a nurse. Lights are used instead of bells. There is complete telephone equipment, the automatic system being used.

Contributions were crucial in realizing the new hospital, especially in meeting construction deadlines. Elizabeth R. Stevens donated $45,000 toward construction of the east wing on condition that citizens of her native Swansea be allowed the same

hospital privileges as Fall River residents. It was named the Stevens Wing in honor of her late philanthropist husband. She also donated $50,000 to help provide free medical care for the Home for the Aged and Children's Home. Carolyn A. Dring donated $10,000 in memory of her father, a prominent Fall River businessman. She stipulated that the library and board room on the second floor be called the Charles P. Dring Memorial Library. On the death that year of Elizabeth M. Borden, Union Hospital's dedicated treasurer, the Borden family donated one hundred shares of Borden Mill stock worth $15,000. Meanwhile, the board of trustees sold the land formerly occupied by the hospital to the Holy Union of the Sacred Heart Academy for $12,000 and moved the old structure to the new site, where it was used for nurses' quarters.

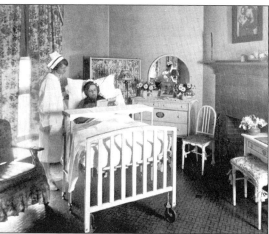

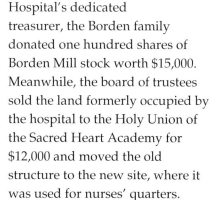
*Private room in the Borden Building, Union Hospital, 1908*

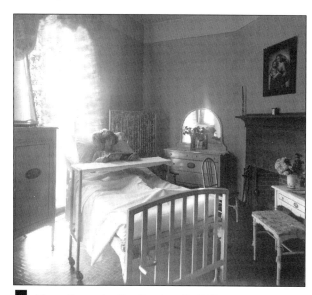
*Almy Room in the Borden Building*

Cont page 15

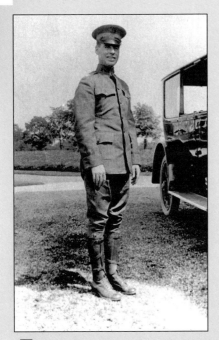

■ *Philemon E. Truesdale, M.D.*

## Philemon Truesdale, M.D.

On a warm June day in 1945, a large crowd of guests mingled on the spacious grounds of Truesdale Hospital as a string quartet of the Boston Symphony played in the background. The occasion was a memorial service for hospital founder Dr. Philemon Truesdale, who had died three weeks earlier.

For most people, Dr. Truesdale's death had been unexpected, although close medical associates had known for years that he had all the symptoms of coronary-artery disease. When they counseled him to take it easy, Truesdale would have none of it. "If you expect me to lie in bed and die, you're crazy," he told a colleague.

Now, as Dr. Warren Atwood; Rt. Rev. Donald B. Aldrich, Bishop Coadjutor of the Episcopal Diocese of Michigan; and Dr. Lucius Kingman spoke of Truesdale's life, mourners summoned their own private memories. They recalled the surgeon, the music lover, the sailing enthusiast, and the entrepreneur. They recalled the visionary and the gambler. They recalled, in short, a man of many facets.

Philemon Truesdale was born in Saint Sherbrooke, Quebec, in 1874, one of five children in a family of English-Irish descent. His father, a lumberjack by trade, brought the family to Fall River in 1879 and settled in French-speaking Flint Village. Young Philemon showed his entrepreneurial bent early when he started a newspaper route and subcontracted the deliveries out to other boys. His territory eventually covered nearly all of Flint Village. Later, at B.M.C. Durfee High School, he stood out academically and played violin in the school orchestra.

In 1894, Truesdale entered Harvard Medical School and paid his way through college by assisting his brother John in his Roxbury flower shop. Even in so modest a business, he prospered by scanning death notices and selling funeral set pieces to the bereaved. After graduation in 1898, Truesdale spent two years as a resident at the Boston Hospital and the Boston Lying-In Hospital, where he became a convert to asceptic surgery. Then he returned to Fall River.

It was in his home town that Truesdale ran afoul of local mores and triggered a rivalry that would fester for more than seventy years. Finding the opportunity to practice surgery practically nil at the new Union Hospital (too many doctors and too few surgery cases), he started up a "storefront" surgical center with Dr. Nathaniel Aldrich. It was an immediate success, and he soon moved to successively larger quarters at the Davol House on Main Street and the former Sacred Heart Rectory. In 1910 Dr. Truesdale built Highland Hospital, an aristocratic neocolonial structure at the end of Highland Avenue overlooking the Taunton River.

None of this endeared him to Fall River's medical establishment, which considered it a breach of etiquette for a doctor to run a private hospital—particularly, it appeared, a successful one. Moreover, Truesdale insisted that physicians practicing at his hospital be approved by the medical staff, which conflicted with Union Hospital's open-staff policy of allowing all physicians access. It reinforced a stereotype of Truesdale as an elitist institution.

In 1914 Dr. Truesdale established the Truesdale Clinic, a prototype group practice, on Rock Street. It was the first of its kind in Fall River. A year later, Highland Hospital went public and was renamed Truesdale Hospital. Over the ensuing decades, the hospital prospered, thanks to the support of the community and philanthropists such as Woolworth cofounder Earle P. Charlton, who singlehandedly contributed $500,000 for a surgery wing in 1927. Charlton never forgot the time Dr. Truesdale and his staff saved his son, Perry, after the youngster's appendix ruptured and peritonitis set in.

In 1929 Truesdale broke new ground with an animated film describing surgery for diaphragmatic hernias. It was the first such film in the United States and opened the door for the use of motion pictures as medical teaching aids. In recognition, the American Medical Association presented Truesdale with its gold medal. But the publicity paled in comparison to the famed "upside-down" stomach operation seven years later, when Fall River was turned into a media circus.

It started when Alyce McHenry, a ten year old from Omaha, Nebraska, was referred to Truesdale for surgical correction of a congenital diaphragmatic hernia. The girl's family was poor, and an anonymous Omaha businessman footed the bills. The national press, still salivating from the Lindbergh trial, sensed a melodrama of Dickensian proportions and descended on Truesdale Hospital en masse. Alyce McHenry was instantly transformed into a combination of Shirley Temple and Little Nell.

Thanks to Truesdale administrator Delight S. Jones, R.N., reporters were barred from the hospital, and the little girl was able to get some rest. On March 4, 1935, Truesdale and his assistants, Drs. Warren Atwood, Cornelius Hawes, and A.H. Miller, commenced the operation. A physician from the New York Academy of Medicine kept the mob of reporters waiting outside informed of progress via telegraph. More than forty medical professionals crowded into the operating room to observe the surgery. Two hours later, it was all over, and Alyce McHenry was able to begin life anew. "This little girl has a pretty serious uphill climb ahead of her," Truesdale cautioned, "and it would be rash to make any predictions." An ensuing headline interpreted the remark to mean: "Alyce Fights Death After Knife's Work."

Dr. Truesdale traced his expertise with diaphragmatic hernias to World War I, when he discovered the new surgical technique while serving with the Yale Mobile Hospital unit in France. Truesdale appropriated and later refined the procedure. During the war, he spent the majority of his time as a battlefield surgeon, rising to the rank of major. After the armistice, he returned home to resume his duties at Truesdale Hospital, which had been ably managed in his absence by Dr. Ralph French. One of Truesdale's strengths, in fact, was his ability to surround himself with top-notch physicians such as Frederick Barnes, William Mason, Delano Ryder, Warren Atwood, Cornelius Hawes, Ralph French, and others.

Despite his many responsibilities, Truesdale found time to live the good life, including ill-fated ventures as a gentleman farmer and ocean yachtsman. In 1935 he bought up several Westport and Little Compton farms, some on the ocean, and tried to develop an exclusive summer colony along the shore. He built bathing pavilions near Warren's Point and on Goosewing Beach. The hurricane of 1938 destroyed them, and the project was abandoned. During the war, he tried to raise Aberdeen Angus cattle to circumvent beef rationing, but government restrictions thwarted his efforts.

In 1936 Truesdale entered the Newport-to-Bermuda yacht race despite having virtually no experience as an oceangoing sailor. His entry was the seventy-five-foot White Cloud, which the *Herald News* described as an "old-fashioned type topsail rigged schooner dressed up with modern equipment, including 3,900 feet of sail." Truesdale's lifelong friend, the dentist W.W. Marvel, told him he was "foolish" to enter the race. "Naturally," Marvel added, "he didn't listen." Marvel wrote of the voyage:

Several hours out of Newport a sudden storm came up and a pretty tough time was experienced to keep the boat afloat and save the supplies. As they neared Bermuda, another fierce storm struck her and the frail boat was dismasted. By the grace of God, they finally arrived at the island under tow but in pretty poor shape.

Marvel once asked the flamboyant surgeon if he was bothered by what people said about him. Truesdale replied, "I don't care what they say as long as they say something. To be ignored is worse." It echoed Teddy Roosevelt's sentiment that "the credit belongs to the person who is actually in the arena, who strives valiantly, who errs and comes short again and again; who knows the great enthusiasms, the great devotions, and who at the worst, if he fails, at least fails while daring greatly." ■

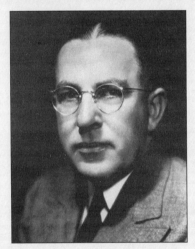

■ *William Mason, MD, past chief of medicine. A model physician, he was respected by his peers and the community. At age ninety-two, he could still be found walking the hospital corridors.*

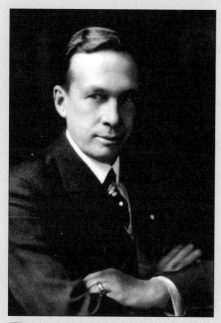

■ *Earle Perry Charlton*

## Earle P. Charlton

When F.W. Woolworth Company tycoon Earle Perry Charlton was born, the Battle of Gettysburg was only days away. And when he died, Herbert Hoover was still president. Yet when Charlton's name is mentioned today, it is almost as if he were still presiding over board meetings.

If wealth can prolong life beyond the grave, then "E.P." Charlton has achieved a degree of immortality. He lives on in the hospital that bears his name and the medical buildings, equipment, and scholarships he has funded. Were it not for his generosity, a substantial number of citizens in the Fall River area and elsewhere might not have lived out full, pain-free lives. The catastrophic illnesses that torment humanity would have had been spared a tenacious adversary.

For all his wealth and sophistication, Earle P. Charlton was not a gentleman to the manner born. He was from rural Connecticut and poorly educated. Charlton began his career as a seventeen-year-old traveling salesman bumping back and forth between Boston and Chicago, selling inexpensive household items out of trunks for a salary of seven dollars a week.

But Charlton was not a garden-variety huckster sporting a bowler hat and cheap suitcase. He was an ambitious young man with an unlimited capacity for hard work. His ability and drive inevitably brought him to the attention of older, successful men such as Sumner Woolworth, Fred Kirby, and Seymour Knox, all of whom owned stores that were prototypes of the five-and-ten-cent chain stores to come.

In 1890 Charlton and Knox became partners, opening their first store on South Main Street in Fall River. Five years and several new openings later, the men split up the business and divided the stores between them. Charlton kept the one in Fall River and began to build his own five-and-ten-cent empire.

Years later, former Fall River store employees would remember Charlton coming to work every day and eating at the lunch counter with the other customers. Sometimes he brought his dog, Asko, with him. Then he would go to his large office on the second floor, where he ran the farflung operations of his thriving company, for another lengthy day. His wife, Ida, helped out by working as a cashier.

Within fifteen years, E.P. Charlton Company Five-and-Ten-Cent Stores had become fixtures not only in New England but all along the West Coast and up into Canada. From California to Quebec and Montana to Nova Scotia, Charlton was a household name. Much of his success was attributable to Charlton's appraisal skills, whether in merchandise or real estate. He reinforced this with a management structure that rewarded only those who produced.

Charlton delegated duty with a minimum of surveillance, but he was quick to deal with transgressors, as this 1910 letter regarding a pilfering manager indicates:

"If you find that this Mr. Ohiser has drawn out, in addition to $28, another $10 in cash, from the till, I want him relieved from management, and take his keys. He is a single man who cannot get along with $20 a week and has to borrow money out of the till. We certainly can get along without him."

Charlton was just as decisive when it came to handling natural disasters. In 1906, notified that the San Francisco earthquake had destroyed the E.P. Charlton store, he issued orders immediately. Within thirty days, the store had been rebuilt at another site and was back in business. It is said to have been the first retail store to resume operations in that devastated city.

That same year, Charlton's son, Perry, suffered a ruptured appendix complicated by peritonitis and was rushed to Philemon Truesdale's small private hospital in Fall River. Dr. Truesdale and his colleagues treated the boy, who recovered, and earned the undying gratitude of the young tycoon. The ripple effects of this seemingly isolated event, which later influenced Charlton in his choice of philanthropies, are still being felt today.

"In his contact with other men," wrote Fall River historian Arthur Sherman Phillips, E.P. Charlton "never assumed any superiority. He had unusual ability to select and enthuse his associates in his business and relied implicitly upon those who would follow his leadership."

In 1912 Charlton merged his fifty-three five-and-ten-cent stores with those of F.W. Woolworth, S.H. Knox, F.M. Kirby, C.S. Woolworth, and W.H. Moore to create a retail chain of 596 stores, the largest in the nation. Within twenty years, the number of stores exceeded two thousand. In the meantime, Charlton became vice president of the chain, now called F.W. Woolworth Company. He sponsored the building of Charlton Cotton Mill, served as a director of B.M.C. Durfee Trust, the city's largest bank, and, during the 1920s, funded a south wing, then a complete surgery wing, for Truesdale Hospital. The cost: half a million dollars.

During World War I, Charlton was appointed a member of the War Industry Board by President Woodrow Wilson and awarded a decoration for his services by the French government. President Calvin Coolidge later selected him to be

president of the Coolidge Fund for the Clark School in Northhampton, Massachusetts. In addition to his government service, Charlton acted as a director of the New Haven Railroad and a trustee of the Massachusetts state-controlled street railroad.

When E.P. Charlton died at his sprawling Westport Harbor summer home on November 20, 1930, he left an estate estimated at $32 million, with nearly $2 million earmarked for charity. It was reportedly the largest estate ever left by a Fall River resident. In Fall River alone, Charlton bequeathed generous endowments to Truesdale Hospital, the District Nursing Association, the Central Congregational Church, the Boys Club, the Y.M.C.A., the Home for the Aged, the Childrens' Home, St. Vincent's Orphan Home, the Ninth Street Nursery, and the Saint John's Day Nursery.

The historical significance of E.P. Charlton's life, according to the historian Phillips, is that "his capital was not inherited nor speculative—it was earned. It took him forty years to amass this vast wealth, and he accomplished what all others had failed to do." ■

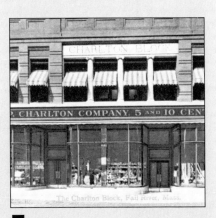
■ *EP Charlton Company*

It had taken six years to reach this point, and the planning committee had done its job well. Union Hospital appeared ready to meet the needs of current generations as well as those to come. And there was room to grow. The new structure was the first of its kind in Fall River to be designed specifically as a hospital. As such, it heralded a national trend. The days of jerry-rigged hospitals in residential homes were over. Emerging technology demanded efficiency in movement and space. It demanded organic design and ease of operation. As a result, doctors came to expect sophisticated work environments. With more professionalism came more fee-for-service patients and a demand for greater privacy in examination rooms and wards. Union Hospital trustees had anticipated this trend in its annual report of 1901. Citizens would find the hospital invaluable, they said, "when an emergency requires ... the skilled treatment of the Hospital, under more favorable conditions than the home may afford."

# Dr. Truesdale Builds His Hospital

*B*y 1910 growing pains seemed to be afflicting all of Fall River. Its population now stood at 119,295, a jump of nearly 15,000 in less than ten years. The textile industry never seemed so strong or the nascent middle class so prosperous. A year later, in fact, President William Howard Taft would personally visit Fall River during its Cotton Centennial, the one-hundredth

anniversary of the city's textile industry. A new world was in the making, and the people of Fall River intended to be part of it. In 1910 aviator Henri Farman flew three hundred miles in eight hours (Glenn Curtis would buzz Fall River crowds a year later), and Barney Oldfield reached the incredible speed of 133 miles per hour in a Benz. The first deep-sea expedition was mounted, and the "weekend" became fixed in American life. Florence Nightingale and Mark Twain died, while Halley's comet shot past earth at a reported speed of forty-three miles per second.

On the local scene, sports fans were rooting for Fall River Baseball Club alumnus Napolean "Nap" Lojoie to beat Ty Cobb for the American League batting title (he did not) and for "The Great White

Hope" Jim Jeffries to beat Jack Johnson for the heavyweight boxing title (he did not, either). Educator and former slave Booker T. Washington reminded a rapt audience at the Central Congregational Church that black America was a nation within a nation. And Earle P. Charlton turned the spade on the new Charlton Mill to begin his venture into textiles.

Charlton was not the only person turning a spade in Fall River that year. The indefatigable Truesdale, seeking more space and a quieter location, built a new hospital at the end of Highland Avenue on a hilltop overlooking the Taunton River. The site, which he purchased from Rudolf F. Haffenreffer for $10,000, was located two miles from the center of the city. When a few of his colleagues suggested that the location was too remote, Dr. Truesdale reportedly said, "If I'm any good as a surgeon, they'll follow me anywhere."

Highland Hospital, as it was named, was designed by Fall River native Parker Morse Hooper and cost $90,000—twice as much as originally estimated. The three-story colonial structure featured open-air verandas, polished wood floors, marble fireplaces, and fine paintings. The exterior was yellow brick of a Flemish bond, while the interior brickwork and firewalls came

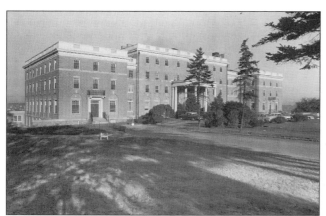

*Truesdale Hospital*

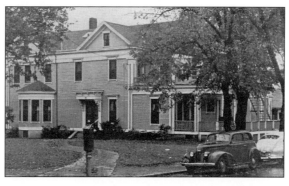

*The Haffenreffer Home, a gift of Mr. and Mrs. Rudolf Haffenreffer, a post-acute nursing home for two decades—it stands across from Union Hospital at Hanover and Prospect streets, and is the current site of Hanover Associates.*

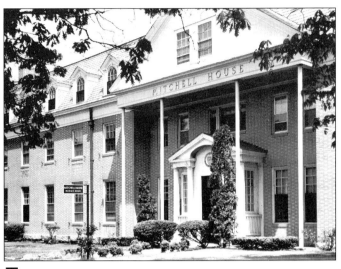

*Mitchell House*

from old ceramic kilns in Somerset. Truesdale wanted a soothing environment, one where "nature offered the sick her marvelous agencies of cure." According to William W. Marvel, a dentist and lifelong friend of Truesdale, the only thing the architect overlooked was closets. Patients had to make do with cubbyholes or armoires.

Initially, nurses occupied the first floor of Highland Hospital, but a swelling patient list began to crowd them out. In 1912, when Dr. Ralph W. French established the hospital's nursing school, Maria Hicks, a grateful former Truesdale patient, funded the construction of Hicks (later Mitchell) House for nursing quarters. Two years later, impressed by Mayo Clinic's innovative group practice in Rochester, Minnesota, Truesdale founded the Truesdale Clinic on Rock Street. "It was felt," he later wrote, "that assembling the doctors' offices in one building would encourage discussions, conferences, study and an esprit de corps."

In 1915 Highland Hospital went public, offering stock and changing its name to Truesdale Hospital. It remained a "closed medical staff" hospital as opposed to Union Hospital, which was "open." The difference was fundamental. Doctors using Truesdale Hospital had to be approved by the Truesdale medical staff. Consequently, they tended to work almost exclusively for the hospital on the hill. Furthermore, Truesdale Hospital was managed by physicians, who were heavily represented on the board of trustees. At Union Hospital, doctors were approved by the board of directors and frequently worked at other institutions such as Saint Anne's and the city hospital. Union Hospital drew a line between business and medicine, entrusting its finances to a board of laymen and limiting doctors to clinical matters. These divergent philosophies would lead to broad, and often unfair, stereotyping by both institutions.

# Meeting the Challenge

*O*f Fall River's social problems, perhaps the most tragic was the infant mortality rate. As late as 1915, it was calculated at 202.3 deaths per 1,000 births. Nothing, it seemed, had changed from the turn of the century, when the rate was 80 percent higher than the national average and approached the combined rates of Chicago and New York. A number of factors, such as poor sanitation, nutrition, and neglect, contributed. Many workers were illiterate and ignorant, not to mention exhausted. But it was the textile industry that laid the groundwork by paying wages so low that living conditions remained substandard, even though both husbands and wives worked. And many wives worked while pregnant. According to Fall River historian Philip T. Silvia, Jr., Portuguese women, more of whom worked while pregnant than women of other ethnic groups, had an appalling infant mortality rate of 299 per 1,000 births.

In addition to infant mortality, there were the usual

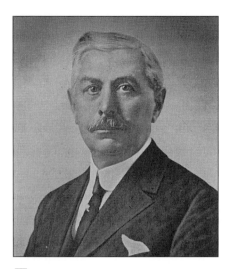

medical problems associated with factory towns: a relentless stream of industrial accidents ranging from contusions to amputations, respiratory ailments such as asthma and pneumonia, and heart disease of various kinds. Salvation would not come overnight, but hope was gaining ground. Illness was no longer simply a cross that had to be borne. It was susceptible to prevention and cure. After all, yellow fever and diphtheria had been virtually eradicated, a skin test for tuberculosis had been developed, and syphilis could now be detected and treated. Furthermore, medical training had improved following the Abraham Flexner Report of 1910, which called for increased clinical experience at the undergraduate

and graduate levels. More doctors were "socialized and educated" in hospital wards. At Union Hospital, nurse training was lengthened to three years in response to tougher criteria by nursing organizations and hospitals. Nurses' duties had broadened considerably, particularly in the arena of preventive medicine. They now visited tenements, schools, and factories, in addition to homes.

In 1912 the U.S. government established the U.S. Public Health Service and the Children's Bureau in a national effort to upgrade medical services. Soon after, the American College of Surgeons incorporated and began the push for hospital standardization. Union Hospital, too, was taking major steps to deal with the most vexing problems of Fall River, despite the fact that the new quarters it had inhabited four years before were now being taxed to the limit. It was a victim of its own success. "The limit of accommodation ... has about been reached," conceded Arthur W. Allen, secretary of the board of trustees. He wryly noted that other businesses were not like hospitals, where "facilities create the demand rather than the demand creating the supply."

The facilities, it seemed, were getting more popular every day. To illustrate, the number of patients admitted annually had soared from 821 in 1908 to 3,316. Most were outpatients, who posted a whopping 451 percent increase. The recent passage of the workman's compensation act locked in the trend. Surgery had nearly doubled—431 to 814 cases—while the number of patient-treatment

days stood at 19,519, of which 3,886 were free. On the other side of the ledger, Allen noted that while the number of patients had risen enormously, costs had risen only 135 percent. And the number of days' treatment per patient and the percentage of deaths remained stable. It was testimony, he said, to the "comparative economy of a large hospital."

That same year, Union Hospital cosponsored the founding of the District Nursing Association, introduced the Well Baby Clinic, and set up clinics throughout the city to dispense pasteurized milk for babies. All would have a positive impact on health in the Fall River area, especially on infant mortality. Union had already inaugurated its social-services department the year before—it was one of the first hospitals in the country to do so—and completed the outpatient department, thanks to funding by Elizabeth Stevens. The hospital also had initiated a free orthopedic clinic to complement X-ray facilities installed in 1909.

But there was more to Union Hospital than medical crusades and eye-popping machines. Union was an extension of community life. Union volunteers—even patients— found themselves performing distinctly nonmedical tasks, such as teaching English to immigrant patients in waiting rooms or wards. "The inability to speak our language is a continual and serious handicap in the relation of the patient and those who would help him in the hospital," reads the 1912 annual report. "It also retards his advancement in the community."

Since 1905 more than ten million immigrants from southern and eastern Europe had flooded into the United States. Those coming to Fall River now were mostly Portuguese. The flow of the previously dominant French Canadians had virtually ceased with the industrialization of their homeland. Still, assimilation went on.

That was a principal reason, among others, that the social-services and outpatient departments were born. Both were groundbreaking ventures. Boston's Massachusetts General Hospital, for example, had opened the nation's first outpatient clinic a scant six years before. Union's social-services department often worked in tandem with the surgical outpatient clinic, tracking down patients who failed to return for follow-up treatment. Most were accident cases from the mills, and many spoke no English. In the Union library, in fact, were books in nineteen different languages representing the ethnic spectrum of Fall River. While visiting the homes of lapsed patients, social workers were able to gather other valuable information, such as family hygiene, the presence of unreported disease, or an infant in need of medical treatment. Social services also operated a convalescent home in Portsmouth for needy patients requiring extended recuperation.

Nurses from the District Nurses Association also paid visits to patient homes, sometimes to assist in delivering babies, other times to report children with congenital deformities, minister to

# Richard P. Borden

When Richard Borden became Union Hospital board of trustees president in 1923, it was as if a providential rain had fallen during a drought. If ever a person was equipped for the task ahead, it was "Dicky" Borden.

It was not the first time Borden had been board president. He had held the post from 1907 to 1913 during a time of rapid economic growth in Fall River. But times had changed. World War I had ended and with it the boom times. Textile mills

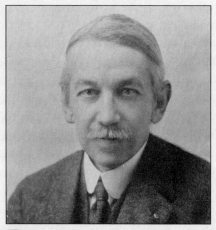

■ *Richard P. Borden, president, Union Hospital, 1907-1913, 1923-1942*

were flowing out of Fall River like a hemorrhaging artery, and only the cheap labor of the South could stanch the wound.

In the meantime, the people of Fall River continued to get sick or injured and to have babies. They continued to require the services of a hospital. It was up to Borden to see that Union stayed afloat, and he did so against daunting odds. Until his death in 1942, Borden helmed Union through municipal bankruptcy and the worst depression in U.S. history. He could be counted on to file the most erudite briefs in Bristol County or to roll up his sleeves in the boiler plant to help chief engineer Manual Carvalho with a problem. He was a hands-on leader.

Borden was born into a prominent Fall River family on April 6, 1865, three days before Lee surrendered to Grant at Appomattox. The Bordens had played key roles in the creation of a steamship line, the Fall River Irons Works Company, American Printing Company, and Richard Borden Manufacturing Company. Borden, who graduated from Massachusetts Institute of Technology and Harvard Law School, forged a reputation as a corporate lawyer.

He probably was as rounded an individual as any who ever came out of Fall River. In the Spanish-American War and again in World War I, Borden served as, respectively, a naval ensign and an army major attached to the general staff in Washington. In addition to his duties at Union Hospital, he was a trustee and director of the American Hospital Association. A patron of the arts, he was a close friend of the painter John Singer Sargent and a regular subscriber to concerts by the Boston Symphony Orchestra.

During the depression, Borden sustained a modest wedge of employment for Fall River by keeping Union Hospital solvent and the Richard Borden Manufacturing Company operating, which he accomplished by loaning his own services and personal credit to the corporation. Richard Borden, a lifelong bachelor, died at Union Hospital on September 23, 1942, after a long illness. ■

the sick, and transport patients to the hospital. The pasteurized-milk clinics, which were funded by Richard P. Borden and Alice Brayton, did much to curtail infant sickness and death by preventing the ingestion of harmful bacteria. The Well Baby Clinic provided outpatient care for mothers of all social levels and remained in operation until 1968.

It was Union Hospital's X-ray facilities that gave the institution a boost in scientific credibility—a phenomenon shared by all hospitals. Since Wilhelm Conrad Roentgen discovered them in 1895, X-rays had fascinated the public, including physicians. The ability to see inside a human body exerted a mystique that still lingers. When X-ray machines were first purchased in the late 1890s, they were seldom used, other than to confirm already completed treatment. Gradually, they came to be valued not only for defining broken bones but in detecting kidney stones and other foreign bodies.

As might be suspected, Union Hospital's X-ray facilities were indispensible from the start and

occupied largely with industrial accidents. In 1911, 277 X-ray plates were used. Two years later, the figure was up to 650 and climbing. "Improvements have been so rapid in this art," reads the 1912 annual report, "as to make our present apparatus out of date ... and negotiations are being made for ... the installation of one which shall be equal to the demands of our people, who content themselves only with the best. The X-ray is one of the most expensive equipment that the Hospital is required to supply." Business was so brisk that in 1914, Dr. Matthew Tennis was hired as a full-time "Roentgenologist." In this respect, Union Hospital was unique. Many hospitals did not get full-time X-ray technicians until years later.

On March 1, 1912, the F.W. Woolworth Co. chain of more than 596 stores commenced operation across the United States and Canada. Within twenty years, the number of stores would quadruple. Fall River's Earle P. Charlton and five other "five-and-ten" store owners had merged their holdings to create the retail giant. Charlton, who owned Fall River's Charlton Mills, contributed fifty-four stores and became a vice president in the new entity. The merger was expected to benefit owners and customers alike through greater cost effectiveness and purchasing power. In years to come, it also would benefit Truesdale and Union hospitals.

# War Comes to Spindle City

*B*y 1917 Fall River was in the midst of what historian Philip Silvia calls "the final burst of dazzling prosperity for the city, the textile industry, capital and labor." America had entered World War I, which meant mill owners were getting lucrative wartime contracts and labor was getting fat raises. Investors were earning dividends of up to 33 percent on capitalization.

Union Hospital, too, was flush with good news. The long-anticipated Stevens Clinic had finally been completed, freeing up the main building for core activities and providing a commodious home for others. It was connected to the main building by an underground tunnel and a heated pedestrian overpass. *Popular Mechanics* magazine gushed over the four-story building and its airy, tiered

■ *Ralph W. French, MD, president, Truesdale Hospital, 1917-1921, 1940-1942*

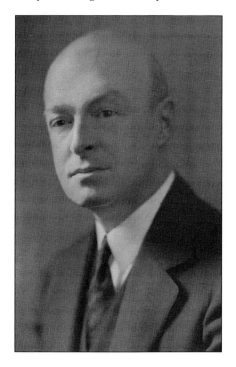

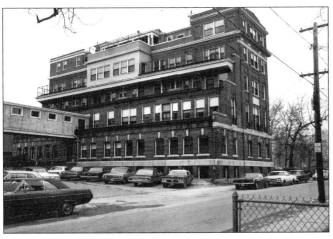

■ *The Stevens Building was built in 1916, with its receding verandas, and heated pedestrian overpass, it was praised in* Popular Mechanics *for being very modern.*

verandas. "It is a structure," said the magazine, "in which many of the most modern ideas of hospital construction have been embodied." Stevens Clinic housed an open and private wards, outpatient clinics, children's ward, X-ray department, and a gym for children's therapy. It was named for its benefactor, Elizabeth R. Stevens.

But as 1917 drifted into 1918, the war began to exact a toll not only on combat forces but on hospitals. Casualties were mounting and doctors and nurses were needed. Many of Union Hospital's best young men and women left to serve in overseas field hospitals or at stateside medical facilities. Philemon Truesdale joined the Yale Mobile Hospital, a select surgical unit, and shipped out to France. During his twenty-month absence, Dr. Ralph French took his place at Truesdale Hospital. With the departure of young staff members, the workload was shifted to senior staff members at both hospitals.

In 1918 Union Hospital also lost the able leadership of its superintendent, Anna Rothrock, R.N., who resigned to devote herself to Armenian relief work. Rothrock had guided Union through a sustained period of growth in which it moved from a 30-bed former private residence to a modern 140-bed main hospital with a separate clinic. Marian Holmes, the assistant superintendent, resigned to serve with U.S. military forces in France.

# The Great Influenza Epidemic

*T*he eighteenth annual report starts off in a funereal tone:

> The year 1918 will certainly go down in the history of the Union Hospital as one of the most trying and difficult since the organization of the institution. The shortage of men on the staff, the demands of the Red Cross Service, which has taken a number of our head nurses and the great shortage of interns are three of the principal reasons.

Another principal reason, aside from the Great War, was the great influenza epidemic, which claimed 21 million dead worldwide and half a million in the United States. So many people were stricken in Lawrence, Massachusetts, that a tent hospital had to be erected on high, open ground to provide isolation and fresh air for the victims. Ambulances ferried them in day and night, while hearses waited for

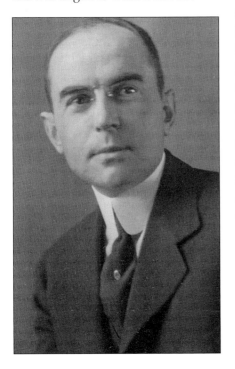

■ *Frederick R. Barnes, MD, president, Truesdale Hospital, 1922-1924*

the doomed. Residents wore masks to work and whispered about the latest friends to die. In U.S. military camps, one in every sixty-seven soldiers died of influenza. It was a melancholy autumn.

Fall River did not escape. At Union Hospital alone, influenza left forty-five dead, including a student nurse named Emma Morill. Of fifty-eight nurses, forty fell prey to the illness. At one point, seventeen of them were incapacitated by illness. Forty-four civilians died out of 109 admitted. The epidemic had started in late August with routine coughs and aches in what was attributed to seasonal change. But the symptoms rapidly escalated to pneumonia and, ultimately, death. Selection was random: The strong died as quickly as the weak. Union Hospital reversed its custom of not accepting contagious patients and threw open ward K in the new Stevens Clinic, reasoning the ward was sufficiently isolated from the rest of the institution. Since city ambulances were burdened with transporting all of the influenza patients, Union's ambulance helped

take up the slack on noncontagious cases, carrying them not only for Union but other facilities as well. The worst months were September through December, but the epidemic did not truly run its course until well after the new year.

In 1919 the Union Hospital annual report alluded to "the unrest which always follows a great war" and its impact on the institution. Numerous staff changes, for example, were made among unnamed "officers and employees," while it was noted that per capita cost for supplies had risen from $2.30 in 1914 to $4.00. In addition, the hospital ran below capacity, with as few as thirty-five beds being used at one point. The number of private patients, ironically, increased from 876 in 1918 to 1,372. This was partly due, the report ventured, to wartime prosperity enabling wage earners, who normally would have "to be content with ward treatment," to afford private rooms. Other hospitals, it added, had undergone the same experience. Union Hospital, like society in general, was feeling the tremors of change. The publication of Lytton Strachey's Eminent Victorians, coming on the heels of ten million war dead, seemed to effectively bury the past.

# Between the Wars

*T*he 1920s have been called the era of flappers and bathtub gin, of Al Capone and Babe Ruth, Bobby Jones and Rudolph Valentino, Lucky Lindy and Damon Runyan. The market was soaring, and even the "little guy" could get rich. Who needed to work? Yet not everyone bought into the get-rich-quick schemes of Wall Street. There were people working and achieving. A number of expatriates, such as writer Ernest Hemingway, preferred to live abroad and avoid what they considered a shallow, materialistic way of life. It was a way of life satirized by Sinclair Lewis in his novel, *Babbitt*. It also was Lewis who wrote the Pulitzer Prize–winning *Arrowsmith*, a look into the life of a medical researcher. Lewis sensed the public's interest in medicine and ran with it.

In fact, there were great things happening in medicine. The war, in its grisly way, had advanced the science of surgery through battlefield expediency. Men were saved who in other conflicts would have died. And many of those men needed reconstructive surgery, which opened up an entirely new field. For the first time, there were fewer deaths from disease—influenza was not a military phenomenon— than from combat. Postwar markers included, the discovery of insulin and penicillin, the development of the "iron lung," and the introduction of the electroencephalograph to record brain waves. The Sheppard-Towner Act, enacted in 1921, helped states combat infant and maternal mortality.

In Fall River, the practice of medicine was a bit more prosaic but no less admirable for the climate in which it was conducted. The wartime prosperity had been, as historian Philip Silvia indicates, an Indian summer. The mills had not expanded, nor had most of them updated their equipment. The strategy was clear: squeeze as much profit out of existing facilities as possible, then leave. One by one, they began packing up and moving south, the railroad cars groaning with equipment. Labor was cheaper there and the cotton closer at hand. When M.C.D. Borden & Sons, one of Fall River's most respected and successful mills, capitulated in 1924, it started a virtual landslide.

If the mills were leaving, illness was not. Union Hospital and its local counterparts were still charged with caring for those unable to care for themselves. Doing so would require resourcefulness, financial help from an increasingly hard-pressed public, and the continued dedication of benefactors. And it would require uncommon leadership. In 1923 Union Hospital got that leadership when Richard P. Borden resumed the presidency of the board of trustees after an absence of ten years. Borden, a corporate lawyer and scion of a prominent Fall River family, had been on the board of trustees since the hospital's inception. He had served as an officer in both the Spanish-American War and World War I. During "Dickey" Borden's

watch, Union Hospital would weather the most turbulent stretches of its existence.

When Borden took the helm, the Fall River economy had not yet faltered, but the shadows were lengthening. Union Hospital was already seeing a rise in free patients—not a new problem, by any means, but one of increasing dimension. Factory "short time" was blamed. Critical cases were climbing, with automobile accidents starting to rival those in the mills. Malnutrition continued to plague low-income families, despite home consultations by social services and the sending of children to summer outings. "Our day is twenty-four hours long," wrote Borden after a detailed description of hospital routine, "and there are no holidays in our year." Union, which had erased a $75,000 debt two years before, now found itself in hock again—this time for $22,000. The cost of running the hospital had more than doubled since prewar days, Borden said, and there was "no relief in sight." Donations and endowments "must increase," he concluded.

In spite of Borden's sober assessment, Union Hospital continued not only to fulfill its role in meeting community needs but to forge ahead. It now had a twenty-four-hour ambulance service, a schoolteacher for convalescing children, and a department of occupational therapy. Union and its rival, Truesdale Hospital, made common cause in organizing blood donors, who were pledged to remain on call (blood could not yet be stored). Union now included insulin in its treatment of diabetics

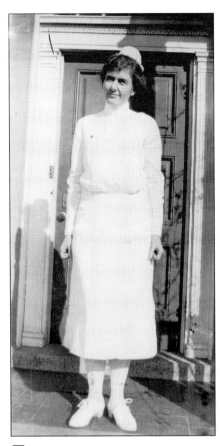

■ *Delight S. Jones, R.N., Superintendent of Nurses at Truesdale School of Nursing, 1928.*

and recently had added a full-time cardiologist and an electrocardiograph to the outpatient department. The "EKG" gained immediate acceptance, fitting into a ready-made format. In 1924 a bronchoscopy and laryngoscopy department was added, followed in 1927 by a diagnostic clinic for cancer. The same year, the Goff Memorial Ward was completed, adding a fifth floor to the Stevens Clinic. In 1928 Union purchased a surgical "radio knife," which cauterized wounds with electrical current. Overall, 3,327 patients were admitted in 1923, with the outpatient clinic averaging 33 patients a day.

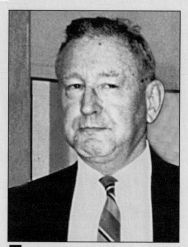

George M. Jackson, administrator, treasurer and trustee

## George M. Jackson

"To George M. Jackson there was nothing more important, after his family, than the hospital and its service to patients. He worked hard at it day and night to promote its growth and development, and most importantly, its mission of service to patients. In 1974, his support of the merger as an influential trustee did much to help make this historical event a reality," reported Frederic C. Dreyer, Jr., his successor.

Jackson was a 33rd Degree Mason, with extensive involvement in masonry regionally and nationally. His involvement in hospitals included regional, state and national appointments. Following his World War I military duty, when he also pursued studies at The George Washington University, in 1938 he began his hospital career as treasurer of Union Hospital in Fall River. In succeeding years he held positions of assistant administrator and administrator. Upon his retirement in 1969, he was elected to the hospital's board of trustees. In 1977 the board of trustees named the board room "The George M. Jackson Conference Room" and declared that the room wherever the board shall meet now and into the future shall continue to be so named in his honor. The designation was made for his "outstanding service to this institution and humanity in various professional and voluntary capacities of treasurer, administrator, trustee and clerk of the corporation."

"His death on July 4, 1980, at the age of 81 left an enormous void with those of us who had the privilege of knowing and working with this remarkable man," Dreyer stated. "He was devoted to his wife, Mildred, daughter, Mary Lou, and family."

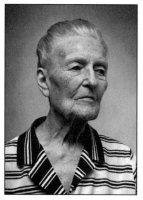

Superintendent of Union Hospital 1942-54, Jennie K. Smithies, in 1972

The school of nursing, too, was thriving, if strapped for space. New quarters were sorely needed. Meanwhile, Union Hospital's Florina F. Goulet, R.N., presented the first report of diseases in terms compatible with international classification, allowing the information to be used by state and civil registrars for vital statistics. As the decade sped by, the name of Jennie K. Smithies began to pop up with regularity—first as an interim superintendent, then as superintendent of the operating department, and later as superintendent of nursing—the first alumnus of the Union Hospital School of Nursing (1916) chosen. By 1929 the nursing school still did not have new quarters, but it had a tennis court, courtesy of Richard P. Borden.

Over at Truesdale Hospital, a south wing was added in 1922, thanks to donations of $25,000 each by Eva McGowen and Earle P. Charlton. Bed capacity increased to one hundred. The gesture by Charlton was completely unexpected, considering that the Woolworth magnate had been out of the picture for several years. "It wasn't until after the war," Dr. Truesdale recalled, "that he became manifestly interested in our ... hospital." In 1927 Charlton again made his presence felt, this time on an unprecedented scale. He funded the entire Charlton surgery wing at Truesdale, which included operating rooms, clinical and pathological labs, research division, radiology department, and twenty private rooms. The price tag: $500,000. Charlton threw in a new ambulance for good measure, a battleship-gray Buick boasting seventy horsepower and a 151-inch wheelbase.

The year before, Truesdale had made an animated film about the surgery used to repair a diaphragmatic hernia. The procedure lowered the mortality rate of such hernias from 90 percent to 30 percent and is said to have been the first medical-education film made in the United States. Truesdale was awarded a gold medal from the American Medical Association for his achievement.

# Fire, Hard Times, and the New Deal

## Chapter Two

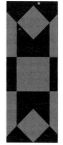

$O$n February 2, 1928, a fire broke out in the Pocasset Mill, which was in the process of being dismantled. It swept through the oil saturated beams and ceilings and outside to nearby buildings. By the time it was contained nine hours later, it had destroyed several city blocks and numerous landmarks. News accounts vividly describe firemen seared by the intense heat while yokes of ice formed around their shoulders. The temperature was zero. Shards of broken glass bedeviled their every step. Before it was over, firefighting units from nearby towns and as far away as Boston had joined in the battle.

With embers burning holes in its top, Union Hospital's ambulance transported victims to all three Fall River medical facilities. Given the timing, the fire could almost be seen as a portent. By 1930, with most of the mills gone and the local economy in shambles, Fall River declared bankruptcy, and the state of Massachusetts took over its finances. In the meantime, both Earle P. Charlton and Elizabeth R. Stevens had died. Breadlines were forming. Union Hospital, as well as Truesdale Hospital, faced an uncertain future.

It was not until 1940 that *The Grapes of Wrath*, a film dealing with the Depression, was made. It was almost as if Hollywood waited until it was safe to examine one of the country's bleakest decades. People had lost their life savings, their homes and sometimes their honor. Fall River residents lived

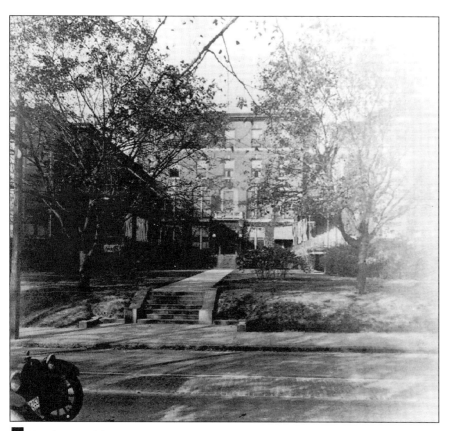

*Borden Building, early 1920s*

with this longer than most. For them, the Depression had come early, when M.C.D. Borden and other mill owners moved out in the midtwenties. By 1932 a quarter of all Fall River residents were on relief, and up to half of them were unemployed. But they were resilient people. They had seen lean times before and survived. This attitude marked Union Hospital as

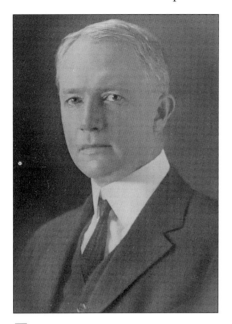

■ *John H. Lindsey, MD, president, Truesdale Hospital, 1930-1932*

well. It would find a way to fulfill its duties as a "charitable institution." That, of course, did not make it any easier.

In 1931 the bequests of Elizabeth R. Stevens and Earle P. Charlton took effect, and Union Hospital felt confident enough to drop the annual fund drive, at least for the time being. It gave the hard—pressed citizenry a temporary reprieve. Though generous, the bequests were supplemental income only, whose dividends were subject to the vagaries of the market. Many times during the 1930s endowment income slipped. As the economy continued to sink, the number of free cases mounted. An accounting in 1933 disclosed 686 free patients, 8,634 free outpatients, and 1,115 partial-pay patients. The city reimbursed hospitals as best it could but still fell far short. In 1935 Union Hospital had 110,719 patient visits at a cost of $61,000. The city reimbursed half of that amount. Fortunately, Union's creditors worked with the hospital, enabling it to meet its medical obligations.

The Fall River General Hospital, a $750,000 structure built in 1924, was not so fortunate and had to trim several departments. Union Hospital absorbed two of them—the outpatient and dispensary services—while Truesdale Hospital took over the ambulance and obstetrics services. St. Anne's, which also offered these services, took up the rest of the

slack. Truesdale, like Union, had to cinch its belt even further with the added tasks. "This hospital," said Charles Davol in Truesdale's 1933 annual report, "has contributed not only directly...but indirectly by the care of many free and part—free patients who otherwise would have been sent to city institutions." Truesdale Hospital also was burdened for several years by

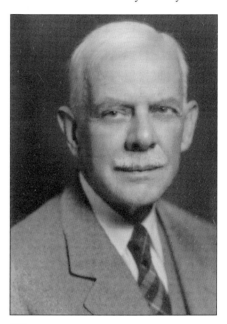

■ *Judge James M. Morton, Jr., president, Truesdale Hospital, 1933-1939*

litigation concerning the pending disposition of Earle P. Charlton's will by the First National Bank of Boston. Eventually, this would be settled by the Supreme Court of the United States.

In 1935 Truesdale Hospital gained national attention when Dr. Truesdale performed surgery on Alyce Jane McHenry, a ten-year-old from Omaha, Nebraska. McHenry suffered from a rare medical condition in which her stomach and intestines pressed through a hole in her diaphragm, causing intense

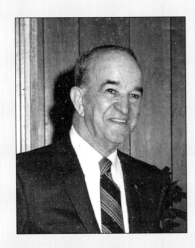

## Manny Carvalho

In 1972 Muriel Mosher did a profile of Manuel "Manny" Carvalho for the Union Hospital newsletter *Pride*. She started off by alluding to him as Union Hospital's version of a Horatio Alger hero. It was not far from the truth.

Carvalho, who was chief engineer at Union for forty years, came up the hard way and made good by dent of ambition and honesty—just like the fictional Alger characters of the nineteenth century. The son of Portuguese immigrants who worked in the mills, he had to quit school at fourteen to watch over his younger siblings. Later he bounced from job to job, all the while taking evening vocational classes in subjects such as mechanical drawing and engineering. What Carvalho lacked in money, he made up for in ambition.

In 1932, at the depth of the depression, the thirty-year-old Carvalho applied for the job of assistant engineer at Union Hospital. Richard Borden, president of the Union Board of Trustees, was so impressed by his references that he hired him on the spot. A year later, he made Carvalho chief engineer. Borden, himself an engineer, often pitched in when Carvalho needed an extra hand. "He was working right along with us whenever he had the chance," Carvalho recalled. "No matter how dirty or how hard the job, he liked getting involved." Carvalho had found a home—and not just figuratively.

For the next thirty-four years, Carvalho and his wife, Albina, lived in a home on the hospital grounds. His daughter, Lillian, who later became the purchasing agent for Union Hospital, grew up there and attended school next door at the Academy of the Sacred Heart. Eventually she married Fred Ferreira, who also worked at Union as an assistant engineer, then staff photographer. Friends of Manny Carvalho recall that he had no quitting time. He frequently could be found checking a gauge or repairing a valve long after working hours. The hospital had become more than just an employer—it had become his life.

As a survivor of the depression, Carvalho was a hoarder, a fixer, and a patcher. Rick Dreyer, who became Union administrator in 1969, recalls that Carvalho could not bear to throw anything away that might be resurrected for later use. That included practically everything. "He had a house next to the hospital crammed full of used parts and equipment," Dreyer says. "I could never really convince Manny that it was more cost-effective to buy new parts and install them before the old ones wore out." On the other hand, it was that kind of obstinate resourcefulness that had kept Union machinery humming through hard times.

As he got older, doctors prevailed upon Carvalho to take some time off for his own health. He bought a summer home in Dighton on the Taunton River. Later he and his wife began making forays to Florida. But he was never more than a phone call away from his beloved hospital. About the time Union consolidated with Truesdale, Carvalho retired—a Union Hospital man to the end. ■

congestion of the heart and lungs. Dr. Truesdale, who was known for his work in the field, performed the so-called "upside-down stomach" surgery in front of some forty prominent physicians, while press from around the country kept a running account of the operation. Today it would be called a media event. The publicity—as expected—was invaluable.

A common thread that runs through the depression years is the repeated generosity of Union doctors and others toward the hospital. With money tight they often dug into their own pockets to buy needed equipment. Dr. George H. Kershaw, for example, donated a Heidbrink portable inhaling machine and a Baxter transfusion set. Later, Dr. Benjamin Leavitt, with friends, purchased two

incubators for the creche. During the same period, an iron lung was donated by an anonymous Union trustee and a therapy tank by the Infantile Paralysis Commission.

Even Union board president Richard P. Borden dug into his own pocket to help furnish supplies. Once he gave the nurses an old green truck to use for general transportation. Jennie Smithies, director of nurses, was chagrined when, a few days later, she saw chief of maintenance Manuel Carvalho hauling trash with it. Smithies soon swallowed her misgivings, reasoning, "Well, the nurses got to use it, too." Times were tough.

Philanthropy, of course, continued to play a crucial role during the uncertain times. In 1934, at the height of the Depression, Ida

S. Charlton, the widow of Earle P. Charlton, established the Ida S. Charlton Fund of $300,000 for Union Hospital. And bequests by the late Elizabeth R. Stevens made possible the opening of Elizabeth House, a nursing residence with classrooms, in 1933. Two years later, the Union Home for Invalids opened, thanks to Mr. and Mrs. Rudolf F. Haffenreffer, who donated not only the property and buildings but renovations as well.(current site of Hanover Associates)

During the depression, the national government took steps to enlarge its role in health care. The New Deal, with its myriad agencies seemingly touching everything in American life, set the tone. The Federal Emergency Relief Administration, for example, supplied funds for rural-health programs, while the Civil Works Administration helped finance disease-control projects. The Social Security Act Grant Funds restored many of the Sheppard-Towner Act's maternal and health-care programs, and the Federal Security Agency brought government health agencies under a single roof. The Farm Security Administration provided group care for poor farmers, migrant workers, and other disadvantaged people through support for medical cooperatives.

It was group care, especially, that attracted public interest. Medicine was becoming ever more sophisticated, with costs threatening to outstrip the individual's ability to pay. Charity was limited. Union Hospital itself

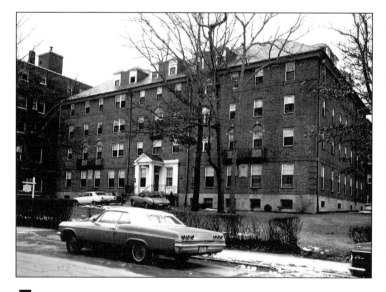

*Elizabeth House, circa late 1960s*

introduced a group hospital plan in 1935 to help defray expenses. For twelve dollars a year, a member received three weeks' care in a private room with no operating-room expenses. Unfortunately, the cost and the premiums cancelled each other out, and the plan was abandoned. It was left to Blue Cross to devise a broad, workable health-insurance plan. By the eve of World War II, 8 percent of all businesses carried such a plan. By the 1950s, almost everyone did.

# Hurricane

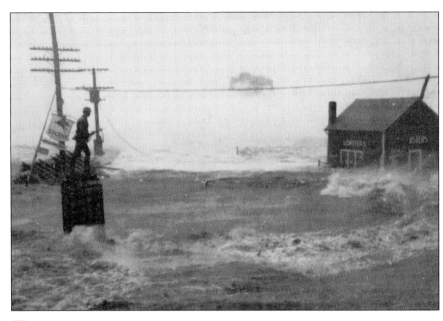

■ *The 1938 hurricane devastated the region, Stone Bridge, Tiverton. Photo courtesy* The Fall River Herald News.

$\mathcal{A}$lmost nobody in Fall River or elsewhere had any warning that September of 1938. The landlocked Weather Bureau in Washington, D.C., wrote it off as a "tropical storm," despite the news that the barometric pressure off the Atlantic coast was the lowest ever recorded; despite word from Miami and the Carolinas that it was moving north with winds up to two hundred miles per hour; despite knowledge that there were high-pressure plateaus offshore and inland that would funnel it into New England; and despite the fact that it would hit at high tide during a period when the moon would be closest to the earth, pulling the tides even higher. After all, a hurricane had not hit New England in 123 years; they always blew out to sea first. And that is what the Weather Bureau forecasted.

Long Island, acting as a breakwater for Connecticut, was the first to get hit by a wall of water so powerful that it registered on a seismograph in Alaska. The mansions of the wealthy were swept away like matchboxes, as people tried to outrun the water in their cars. The hurricane roared unimpeded into Rhode Island, creating a one-hundred-foot tidal wave that raced up Narragansett

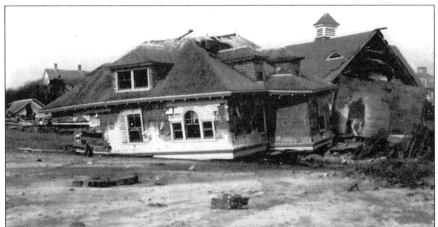

■ *The Charlton estate "carriage house" at Westport Harbor was severely damaged by the 1938 hurricane. Nearby, the beautiful brick home of Ruth and Frederick Mitchell was so badly damaged, it had to be destroyed. Photo courtesy* The Fall River Herald News.

Bay and crushed the docks at Providence. By the time it subsided, Providence lay under thirteen feet of water. Fall River and surrounding towns tasted the violence, too. Power was knocked out, and people took shelter where they could. Dr. Roger Violette, a young intern at Union Hospital, delivered a baby by candlelight. And an out-of-town couple found food and shelter in Union. They later reciprocated by bestowing the gift of an Albee Comper table, used in orthopedic surgery. It was the first of its kind in the city.

The hurricane demolished nearly everything in its path. By the time it was over, seven hundred people had been killed and more than twice that many injured, and sixty-three thousand homes had

been lost. Damage was estimated at $3.6 billion. In Westport Harbor, the names of estates damaged or destroyed read like a who's who of the southeast Massachusetts social register: Charlton, Mitchell, Atwood, Truesdale, Brayton, Durfee, French, Waring, Davol, Walsh, Hawes. The list went on. Strangely enough, few people outside of New England seemed aware of the event—partly because damage to communication lines hampered and delayed media coverage, but mostly because all eyes were on Munich, where Neville Chamberlin was negotiating for "peace in our time." When the pact was signed, everyone breathed a huge—and premature—sigh of relief.

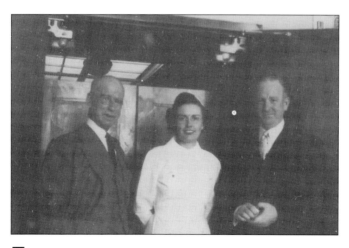

■ *Dr. Truesdale, Hilda Smith and Dr. Gallery*

# Wartime

*I*n 1941 things were picking up, even in Fall River. The war in Europe had stimulated the economy and orders were flowing into the local Firestone Rubber & Latex Products Company plant. In addition, a fledgling garment industry had sprung up in the past few years to complement the few remaining textile mills. The garment jobs paid less than the mills, but any work was welcome. After all, prices kept going up. Chuck roast was seventeen cents a pound now, Porterhouse twenty-five cents a pound, and three pounds of Macintosh apples cost nineteen cents. A high-ticket item such as a stuffed chair went for $24.50.

That year Dr. Karl Lowenthal was appointed full-time pathologist at Union Hospital, replacing recently deceased Dr. James Walsh, who had serviced area hospitals on a commission basis. In a letter to Dr. Lowenthal, Union Hospital board president Richard P. Borden stated the terms of his employment: $83 a month, plus 50 percent of all lab fees, to include use of lab equipment and personnel for nonhospital (Lowenthal's private) patients. Also, permission to charge and collect fees "as you deem necessary for your private account." Topping it off, two weeks' vacation. "If the above comes to less than $5,000 per annum," Borden continued, "the hospital will make up the difference."

Union Hospital kept busy in 1941, with 680 more patients and 3,982 more patient days than the previous year. The annual report voiced concern that the hospital, beset with rising costs, would not be able to meet the future needs of an expanding population, as reflected in the number of babies (623) delivered over the year at Union. The report ruminated about the lack of young women of "high character and educational background" available for nurse training. A college education might be of more value, it groused, because "it would undoubtedly be easier and afford more opportunity for pleasure, which seems to be a major consideration these days." Amid matters of such gravity, staffers seemed to have all but forgotten the recent earthquake that rattled local windows but little else. They did not forget the fire at the Firestone plant that broke out in October and caused an estimated $12 million in damages.

On December 7, Fall River was rocked by a quake of another kind. "Hawaii Suffers 3,000 Casualties, with Nearly 1,500 Persons Dead; Battleship Capsizes In Harbor," read the *Fall River Herald News*. Japan had attacked Pearl Harbor. Local loom fixers cancelled a scheduled walkout "in the interests of national defense," and the state guard was mobilized to protect the Brightman Street and Slades Ferry bridges, together with

bridges at New Bedford and Newburyport. Almost immediately, doctors began leaving Union Hospital for military service, no doubt rekindling memories in older physicians who stayed behind. Nurses, too, left to join the Cadet Nurse Corps and various service branches. A letter dated May 12, 1942, from Dr. M.N. Tennis to Madison F. Welsh, clerk of the board of trustees, relayed a request from Dr. G. R. Horan for a "leave of absence for the duration." Tennis recommended approval.

That same year, Richard P. Borden died, leaving behind a legacy of astute and compassionate leadership through the most trying years of Union Hospital's existence. Borden had served two terms as board president, totalling twenty-five years and forty-four years on the board itself. He was succeeded by John S. Brayton, whose grandfather and father had served as president and trustee respectively. In other staff changes, Jennie Smithies was appointed superintendent of Union Hospital, while George Jackson, who had come aboard as treasurer in 1938,

added business manager to his title.

During the war, Truesdale Hospital became a major blood collector for the armed forces. It was one of nine Massachusetts hospitals so designated. By the end of 1943, the Red Cross had collected a cumulative total of 5,652,000 pints. During that year, an infantile paralysis epidemic in the United States killed 1,200 people, many of them children, and crippled hundreds more.

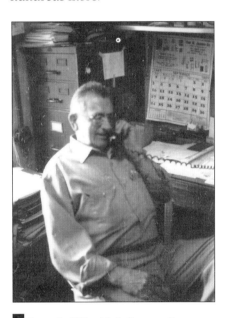

Joseph "Blackie" Boyer, Sr., chief of engineering and maintenance, Truesdale Hospital, 1967

Although the war slowed medical research, work still went on. Streptomycin was discovered, penicillin was used to successfully treat chronic diseases, and the first "blue baby" operation was performed. By the time the war ended, a host of diseases, including smallpox and cholera, had been eradicated. Many others, such as tuberculosis, influenza and VD, had been greatly reduced.

In 1945 Union Hospital was involved primarily in restoration, renovation, and replacement. Among other projects, an air conditioner was installed in the operating room, new surgical instruments were purchased to replace old ones, and the "long unused" Goff Memorial floor was remodeled into a large, airy classroom with lecture hall.

Several doctors and nurses returned from war duties, and others were expected to follow soon. "It is hard to realize," the annual report read, "that in spite of war conditions, when other hospitals are being forced to curtail services to their community, the Union Hospital has increased its services, as reflected by the increased number and daily average of patients." That May a battered Germany surrendered. In August Japan bowed to the atomic age. That year, Philemon Truesdale died, ending a phenomenal career— but not the institution he had founded. ■

# Post War Boom

*Chapter Three*

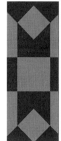

*W*ith the war over, the United States assumed the mantle of medical leadership in addition to its other duties as a global power. America played a leading role in rebuilding the devastated medical facilities of Europe and its former colonies. Government and private groups, such as the Red Cross, were involved, while funds also were channeled through the World Health Organization, an arm of the newly formed United Nations. Public interest in medicine was never higher, the war having played a major role in raising the level of awareness. The big Oscar winner in 1946, for example, was *The Best Years of Our Lives*, an uncommonly adult movie about three exservicemen adjusting to civilian life. One of the actors, Harold Russell, won an Oscar for his superb portrayal of a double amputee. Russell was not, strictly speaking, an actor but a real life veteran whose arms had been destroyed by fire.

In 1946 several other events occurred that made an impact on medicine and the American public. Dr. Benjamin Spock published his Baby and Child Care, a book that would influence two generations of parents; the Communicable Disease Center was established in Atlanta; and the Hill-Burton Act, which provided federal funding for health facilities in small communities, was passed by the U.S. Congress. On a minor but significant note, monkeys were successfully vaccinated against poliomyelitis, raising cautious

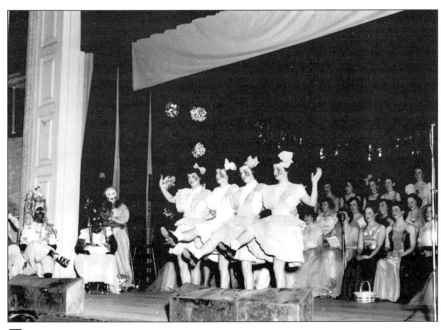

*Follies dancers, circa late 1940s, Union Hospital*

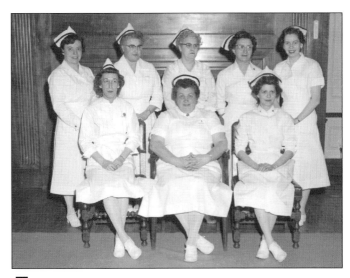

Head Nurse Supervisors Group, Truesdale 1957: (first row) Vivian Potvin (Horton); Margaret Clayton (McDonald); Yvette Lafond (Chase); (second row) Ruth Hurley; Edna Roberts; Emily Bellman; Anne Lewis; and Eileen Gleeson

hopes that the same might be done with humans.

In Fall River, the Union and Truesdale hospitals were gearing up for the postwar world. Technology would alter their approach but not their personas. Over the next twenty years, the widespread use of health-insurance programs, such as Blue Cross, would drive up admissions, while inflation would drive up costs. And the sounds of accents would punctuate the wards as foreign interns flooded in, partly to compensate for the lack of American medical students. In 1956 the Union, Truesdale, and Saint Anne's nursing schools began sharing Bradford Durfee Technical Institute for the teaching of physical and biological sciences, a harbinger of things to come.

Despite medical advances, the Union and Truesdale caseloads still were formidable. If the postwar era brought with it unparalled affluence, it also brought new threats to health. America had a corner on the market, and a generation that had been raised during the depression and fought a global war now intended to enjoy life. Television replaced radio as the preferred medium. In 1950, for example, there were 1.5 million sets in the United States. The following year, ownership had exploded to 15 million. TV brought with it not only the evening news but a more sedentary way of life. Added to that were rich foods, cigarette smoking, and a "three-martini-lunch" mentality. The result was a rise in degenerative diseases usually associated to old age but now also linked to life-style. There was increased incidence of cancer, stroke, heart disease, and diabetes.

If people could not be persuaded to be more moderate, technology could at least alleviate, sometimes even cure, their ailments. Both Union and Truesdale hospitals saw the future and moved ahead. In 1947 the American

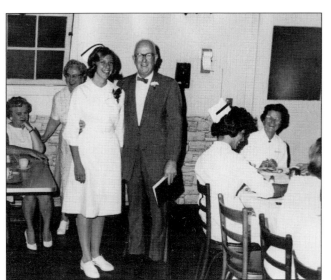

Dr. Daniel Gallery and Irene Boykin, a new graduate of Truesdale Hospital's Nursing School, circa 1960s.

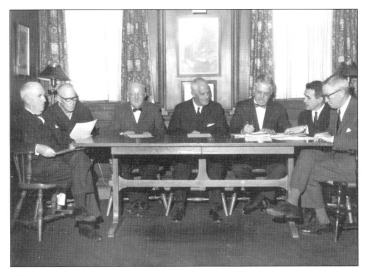

Truesdale Hospital Board of Directors: John B. Cummings, Esq.; Frank Coolidge (who was at that time a patient in the hospital); James Fitzgerald; Albert G. "Bud" Pierce; Gilbert van Blarcom; Joseph A. Faria; Philip Brayton

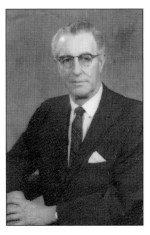

Charles M. Moran, president, Union Hospital, 1961-1974 Under his board leadership, the Union Hospital expanded and modernized its facilities and services. As trusted and capable board leader, Mr. Moran earned the respect and confidence of several generations of trustees.

Cancer Society of Massachusetts donated a $6,000 high-voltage X-ray machine to Union in memory of Dr. Thomas Almy, recently deceased president of Union's medical staff. Union doubled the size of its X-ray department the following year and installed additional equipment at a cost of $12,000. In 1955 the Jacob Ziskind Laboratory opened at Union, thanks to the Ziskind estate, which generously gave the hospital $100,000 to build the clinical and pathological facility. Jacob's brother, Abraham, was an active Union board trustee.

In 1961 Union became one of the first hospitals in the country to use a television fluoroscope, a state-of-the-art diagnostic tool with remote controls and a 35-mm movie camera. The fluoroscope used 90 percent less radiation than other tools. In 1954 Truesdale Hospital introduced a special room equipped for both diagnostic and therapeutic use of radioisotopes, a cutting-edge technology. Two years later, it opened an isotope lab.

New construction, headed up by Charles Moran, chairman of the Union Hospital building committee, proceeded apace with technological innovation. In 1952 a tunnel between the Main and Stevens buildings was completed. Seven years later, Union dedicated the Brayton Building, a 46,436-square-foot structure featuring sixty additional private rooms (expandable to ninety) at a cost of

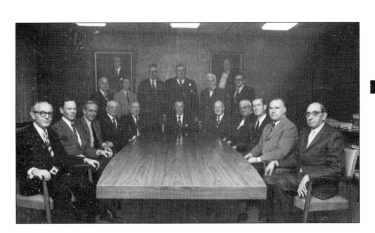

Union Hospital Board of Directors: (standing) Dennis A. Toomey; George Bounakes, MD; Forest Cook; Thomas F. Higgins, MD; Daniel L Mooney, MD; Frederic C. Dreyer, CEO; (seated) Myer N. Sobiloff; Henry Ashworth; Bertram A. Yaffe; Madison F. Welsh; George M. Jackson; Charles M. Moran, president; William M. Hoban; Lawton S. Brayton; Paul V. Stevens; Francis T. Meagher, Esq.; and Louis F. Fayan

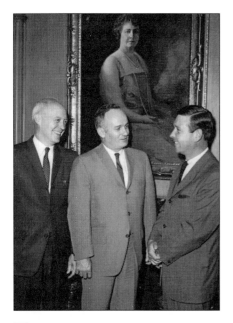

E. Vernon Bradbury, treasurer;
Robert S. Murray, president;
and F. Bliss Winn,
administrator, in the Ida S.
Charlton Library at Truesdale,
circa early 1970s

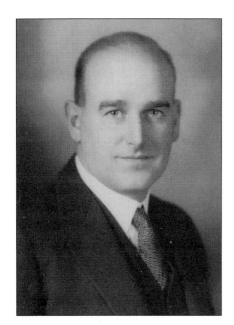

John S. Brayton, president,
Union Hospital, 1942-1961

$1.7 million. A southern extension of the new building containing offices, eating facilities, obstetrical department, and twenty-six semiprivate beds, was completed in 1962 with a price tag of $1.6 million. Hill-Burton provided $300,000, but the depleted building fund had to borrow nearly $700,000. In 1959 Truesdale Hospital added an east wing, providing seventy more beds and increasing its bed capacity to one hundred sixty-nine.

During the postwar years, individual contributors, past and present, continued to exert a heavy influence on the affairs of both hospitals. A retrospective look at endowment funds given to Union Hospital by Frank and Elizabeth Stevens disclosed they had given a total of $879,129.34. There also remained, among others, the Ida Charlton Fund of $300,000, given to a struggling Union Hospital in the depths of the depression. In 1955 Union board president John S. Brayton, in conjunction with his

brothers Flint and Anthony and sister Edith B. McDowell, donated their six-and-a-half-acre Brayton estate, which was adjacent to the hospital. And, as always, Truesdale Hospital enjoyed strong support from the Earle P. Charlton family. In 1949 Charlton's daughter, Ruth Mitchell, donated the Ida S. Charlton medical library, complete with furnishings salvaged from the Mitchell home, which was destroyed by the 1938 hurricane.

The postwar era was marked by medical triumphs both locally and on the national scene. In 1951 the heart-lung machine was invented. A year later, the first open-heart surgery was performed. And in 1955 Jonas Salk's polio vaccine was approved for general use, virtually eradicating a dreaded disease. In 1963 Dr. Michael DeBakey used an artificial heart during surgery.

By Union Hospital's fiftieth anniversary, infant mortality had fallen to 23 deaths per thousand births, a reduction of 179 per

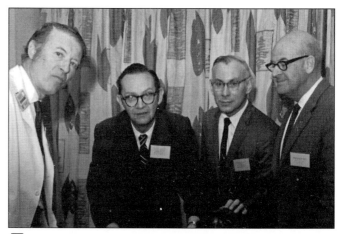

The John C. Corrigan Memorial Foundation brought
noted speakers to Union Hospital. Eugene A. Field,
MD; William J. Grace, MD (speaker), professor of
clinical medicine at New York University Medical
College and director of medicine at St. Vincents
Hospital Medical Center, New York City; Albert
Resnick, MD, and Rupert von Trapp, MD.

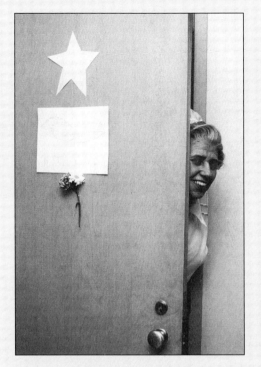

## Eleanor E. Presbrey

One of Eleanor Presbrey's earliest memories was of being a nine-year-old patient at Union Hospital. She was a little frightened at first, especially of Jennie Smithies, the formidable nurse who would later become Union superintendent and a professional colleague of Presbrey's. But as the young Presbrey's hospital stay lengthened—she would remain three weeks—she came to stand in awe of the nurses as they efficiently and cheerfully went about their business. She began to think about nursing as a career.

Presbrey did not get much encouragement from home, even from her two uncles, who were physicians. Get a college education, her family told her. That is more important. After graduating from Fall River's Durfee High School, Presbrey earned a bachelor's degree in sociology and psychology from Wheaton College in Norton, MA. Afterward, she dutifully worked as a service representative for New England Telephone Company until World War II

erupted and—as in the case of other people—gave her an out. That was when she joined the Cadet Nurse Corps and began her studies at Johns Hopkins University.

Suddenly, the repressed nurse took fire. "We all worked harder than we ever had in our lives," Presbrey recalled in a *Pride* article, "and we looked forward to the next day to working again. We had the finest professors and doctors to be found." Because the war had drained hospital personnel, Presbrey and her classmates were given unusual opportunities for growth, particularly in clinical matters. After receiving a B.S. degree from Johns Hopkins, Presbrey spent four years as director of nurses at Virginia's Roanoke Memorial Hospital before coming to Union in 1951 as director of nursing services and director of the Union Hospital School of Nursing.

During twenty-six years at Union and Union-Truesdale, Presbrey pushed hard to improve educational and professional standards. She served as a bridge between traditional and modern nursing. In the 1950s, she waged a five-year campaign of improvement that culminated in the Union School of Nursing receiving accreditation from the prestigious National Nursing Accreditation Association. During this period, Presbrey earned a master's degree in nursing-service administration from Boston University. It took her four years to do it, working full-time. Later, she became a clinical professor in BU's school of nursing.

Presbrey is remembered as a confident woman with a quick, decisive

stride who stood up for her beliefs yet was the ultimate team player. Former boss Rick Dreyer recalls that sometimes "she might not agree with what I said, but I could always trust that she would give her all to support what had to be done, and to me personally." Sometimes, he quips, it was Presbrey who prevailed. Those who knew her paint an affectionate portrait of a top nurse who was dependable, savvy, and always human. Presbrey represented not only the best in nursing tradition but the farseeing nature of Charlton's leadership.

At her retirement, she predicted that nursing and hospitals would involve more administrative entanglements and government red tape. "To lead, you have to know how to cope," she said. "You can't just walk away from bureaucratic problems." ∎

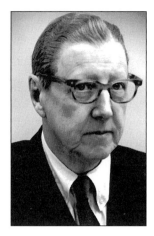

*John C. Corrigan, MD, Union Hospital chief of medicine during the 1960s was often called the "physician's physician." He attended all board of trustees meetings during the 1950s and 1960s.*

thousand from 1915. Life expectancy was close to seventy years, contrasted to forty-nine at the turn of the century. All the while medical education was growing exponentially. In 1951 Fall River native Eleanor E. Presbrey joined Union Hospital as director of nursing. Presbrey, who had a master's degree from Boston University, worked hard to strengthen training and nursing qualifications, as well as to promote nursing as a profession. Eventually, the Union Hospital School of Nursing won accreditation from the National Nursing Accreditation Service, climaxing a five year campaign led by Presbrey. In 1963 Dr. John  C. Corrigan, M.D., established the Union Hospital Department of Medical Education. The postgraduate program, which targeted general practitioners, began a continuing- education

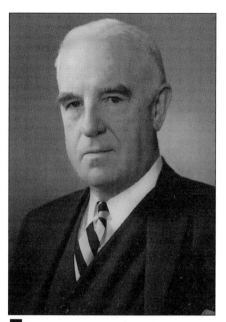

*John B. Cummings, Esq., president, Truesdale Hospital, 1953-1965*

program that soon branched into specialized fields.

Shortly after World War II, a persistent rumor began to circulate in Fall River medical circles. It

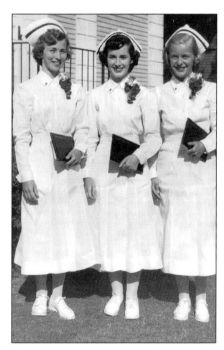

*Truesdale Hospital Nursing School graduates 1950: Geraldine Hopkins, Shirley Audet, and Barbara Lucas.*

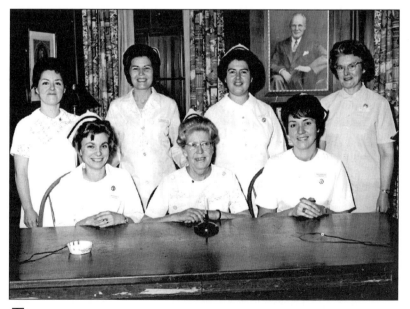

*Truesdale head nurses in the Mitchell Room, circa early 1960s: (seated) Martha Santos, Dolores "Del" Crispo, B. Nikinas; (standing) Marilyn Bradford, Virginia Zillis, Mary Ann Wordell and Catherine Hoefling*

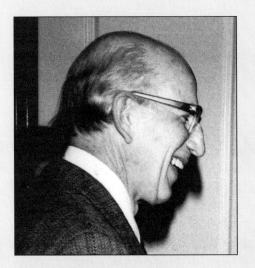

## Frank J. Lepreau, M.D.

One does not hear much anymore about the Albert Schweitzers and Tom Dooleys of the world—probably because they are in short supply. Admittedly, things are more complex than when they practiced their no-frills medicine forty years ago in the poverty-ridden backwaters of Africa and Asia. Still, there are a few altruistic souls willing to sacrifice hearth and home in an attempt to relieve the suffering of disadvantaged fellow humans. Former Charlton physician Frank J. Lepreau is one of them.

Dr. Lepreau, who now tends to the elderly at Cardinal Medeiros Residence in Fall River, can look back on a life rich with service to others. He can take satisfaction in having done "the right thing." Hundreds of poor people in Haiti and eastern Kentucky will vouch for that. It is because of him that many are alive and functioning.

In 1964 Dr. Lepreau decided to volunteer for service in Haiti. During his nine-year tour, the former president of the Truesdale medical staff worked for the sum of $6,000 on average a year. His patients often gave him chickens, goats, fruits, and vegetables in return for services rendered. He did not spend his time on the island alone but was accompanied by his wife, Miriam, and two of their five children. Living conditions were spartan, but the adventurous family made the best of it. As the only chest surgeon on the island, Lepreau performed nearly five hundred lung resections during his stay. In Haiti, tuberculosis is rampant. Also prevalent are typhoid, dysentery, and diphtheria—diseases all but eliminated in the United States. Lepreau worked at Schweitzer Hospital, an appropriately named institution with 160 beds and fourteen physicians. Nevertheless, it was not able to adequately care for the flood of patients, some of whom traveled up to one hundred miles on foot seeking help. It fell to the outpatient department to take up the slack. In one year alone, the OP treated some 85,000 patients. While serving in Haiti, Dr. Lepreau developed expertise regarding lockjaw and wrote a clinical paper that was published in the prestigious British medical journal, Lancet.

Lepreau, a graduate of Dartmouth College and Harvard Medical School, also spent 1974 in eastern Kentucky amid the coal miners of Appalachia. Conditions, he observed, were as primitive as in Haiti. His transportation was a four-wheel-drive Jeep, in which he used to scramble up dry creek beds on house calls. He also descended four miles into the mines to observe health conditions. As surgeon and medical director of the Frontier Nursing Service, Lepreau was heavily involved in training nurse practitioners, who performed the bulk of medical work in the area. He wrote a guidebook for nurse practitioners titled Medical Directives for the Frontier Nursing Service. Among other honors, Dr. Lepreau is the recipient of Fall River Exchange Club's Golden Deeds Award for his service to humanity. ∎

## Cerebral Palsy Clinic

In January 1948, Fall River resident Mrs. William Goldman approached William Kenney, M.D. about the special needs of children afflicted with cerebral palsy. Mrs. Goldman's son, Mark, required therapy in Boston several times a week. Dr. Kenney joined with several other Fall River residents in March 1948 to form a corporation for the purpose of diagnosing, treating, and generally helping to solve problems associated with the disease. Dr. Kenney became its medical director and driving force.

The Truesdale Hospital donated a home located across from the hospital at 218 Calvin Street. Funding was provided by Easter Seals; Jacob Ziskind, a local philanthropist; the United Way; and Azab Grotto, a Masonic order.

The Training Center, as it was called, offered speech and occupational therapies, group activities, special education and orthotics. Patients paid on a voluntary basis. The programs became so popular that in 1963, the center broke ground for a new building at 263 Stanley Street.

In 1970 the Cerebral Palsy Training Center was accredited by the Commission on Accreditation of Rehabilitation Centers, one of only thirty-five in the country.

By the 1980s there were many other programs available for people with cerebral palsy and similar conditions. In 1982 the center's board of directors sold the building to Truesdale Clinic, Inc. ∎

concerned consolidation. In 1949 the Union Hospital annual report suggested that Fall River's hospitals might be joined. A number of professionals believed efficiency would be better served and duplication avoided with fewer hospitals. Speculation centered around the Union and Truesdale hospitals as the institutions most likely to merge. But fifty years of competition made this a volatile proposition. Union and Truesdale made common cause easily enough when taking part in noncompetitive projects. A joint fund-raising drive in 1956, for example, yielded a record $1,350,000. Union received two-thirds of the money, based on its larger size. At one point, Union board trustee Charles M. Moran actually met with John B. Cummings, Truesdale board president, to discuss the possibilities of consolidation. Both were strong minded men with intense loyalties. When Moran returned from the meeting, he muttered a cryptic, "Let's dig a hole," meaning Union should get on with construction and its own agenda. There would be no coming together. Despite the finality of Moran's tone, the ideal of consolidation would not go away. Time and events would see to that.

By 1964 Union Hospital was treating half of all free cases in Fall River—a result, in part, of the closing of Fall River General Hospital. At that time, Union, Truesdale, and Saint Anne's had been obliged to assume responsibility for the city institution's stranded patients. Union, as the biggest hospital, took

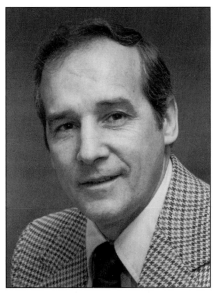

■ *Edward R. Boyer has been employed for forty-five years, thirty years as director of engineering and maintenance. Rick Dreyer says, "Of all the trustees, volunteers, and employees I have had the privilege of knowing and working with, there has never been a more dedicated, dependable, trusted, loyal employee of this institution than Ed Boyer."*

on the lion's share. Free cases at Union had doubled since 1955, with emergency-ward visits tripling since 1960. Yearly admittance now topped ten thousand. Amid the postwar boom, the old challenges remained. With the coming of Medicare and Medicaid, they would be transformed into new challenges. ∎

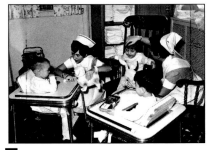

■ *Nurses entertain children, circa early 1960s*

# Toward a New Age

# *Chapter Four*

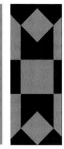

*N*ineteen sixty-five was a good year for America, despite the Watts riots, the buildup in Vietnam, and a blackout in the Northeast that briefly left thirty million people without electricity. The country was riding the crest of a postwar boom that had come to be taken for granted. It seemed everyone was getting a piece of the action this time around. Mortgages were 5 percent, gas went for a quarter a gallon, and more people than ever were earning college degrees, thanks to prosperity, low tuition, and the GI Bill. Baby boomers toured Europe in beat-up VWs while their parents flew to the Caribbean or Las Vegas, where they caught Frank Sinatra's act. In 1965 "It Was a Very Good Year" and "A Hard Day's Night" could still be heard on the same radio station.

Scientific achievement proceeded apace, with astronaut Edward White floating outside of Gemini 4 for twenty-one minutes, only a synthetic umbilical cord tethering him to earthly concerns. And Bell Laboratories researchers Arno Penzias and Robert Wilson used powerful antennas to pick up "space noise"—radio waves, actually—from the Milky Way. Their discovery reinforced the "big bang" theory of an expanding universe. In 1965 conventional films such as *The Sound of Music* and *Doctor Zhivago* were scoring with moviegoers, while the Beatles' "Help" anticipated MTV by twenty-five years.

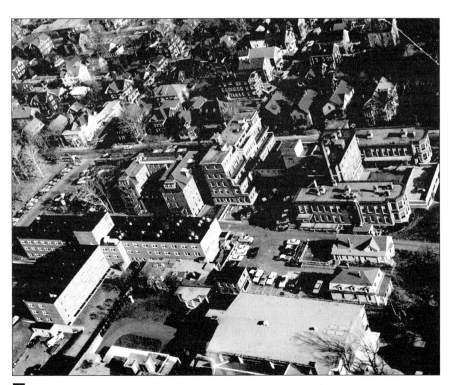

*Union Hospital, taken by Alfred "Freddie" Ferreira from Dr. Joseph Shea's airplane circa 1960s.*

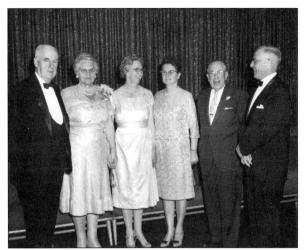

John B. Cummings, Katherine Thompson, Grace De Andrade, Ann Marin, William Mason, MD, and Hayden Deaner (administrator) attend a social event at Truesdale Hospital.

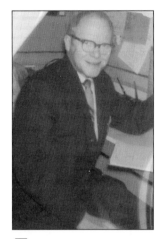

Gordon Stokes, MD, Truesdale Hospital

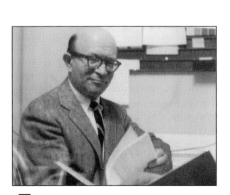

Samuel Brown, MD, Truesdale Hospital

Advance elements of the counterculture were just beginning to arrive but not in numbers sufficient to cause alarm. Long hair, illegal drugs, antiwar protests, bra burnings, and campus takeovers were hovering like attack helicopters just over the horizon. Meanwhile chunks of the past were breaking loose from the firmament. Winston Churchill, the dashing young adventurer who had captivated turn-of-the-century Fall River society, died at ninety-one. He was joined that year by broadcast pioneer Edward R. Murrow, author W. Somerset Maugham, statesman Adlai Stevenson, and former Vice President Henry Wallace.

A few prescient souls could be forgiven the feeling that change was in the air. But it was change that would come from all levels and not just the street. President Lyndon Baines Johnson was about to introduce America to a genuine sixties revolution. It was called Medicare, and it would spearhead his Great Society juggernaut. Along with its twin, Medicaid, it would change the face of American medicine.

It was not as if the national government had not been involved with medicine before. In fact, the government had been making inroads for thirty years. It began during the depression when a down-and-out economy prompted the creation of New Deal agencies to provide rural medical cooperatives, disease control-programs, and maternal-health programs. By World War II, the government boasted an influential role in the distribution of health benefits.

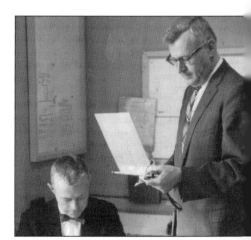

Drs. Leslie Schroeder and Norman H Truesdale Hospital

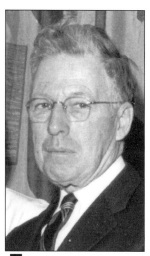

Ernest M. Fell, MD, author of uncompleted manuscript, "A Short History of Union Hospital in Fall River."

In 1945, a month after the Japanese signed surrender documents on board the battleship *Missouri*, President Harry Truman proposed a comprehensive health-care program for the nation in his first message to Congress. It was wide-ranging and included stepped-up construction of hospitals, expansion of health services, and more medical education and research—all supported by federal funds. Truman even proposed prepayment for medical care and protection against loss of wages from sickness or disability, items the American Medical Association staunchly opposed.

Nevertheless, much of Truman's proposal took root, most notably the Hill-Burton Act of 1946, which provided matching funds to states for hospital construction, with emphasis on rural communities. Hospitals receiving funds were assured government would not interfere in their operations—and it did not. One observer called it "an almost ideal working relationship between federal and state governments." The federal government also began long-term channeling of funds for basic and clinical research to the National Institutes of Health, the National Science Foundation, and the Atomic Energy Commission. By 1967 contributions to the NIH exceeded $1 billion annually.

Early proponents of government support for medical research were physicians Paul Dudley White and Michael DeBakey. White, a Boston cardiologist, gained fame in 1955 when he was called in as a consultant during President Eisenhower's heart attack. He used his moment in the spotlight to push for more government funding. In

1964 DeBakey, professor of surgery at Baylor University in Texas, headed a federal commission to develop, in his words, "a realistic battle plan" for conquering heart disease, cancer, and stroke. DeBakey noted that even though the gross national product was spiraling upward toward $1 trillion, America was investing only $1 billion a year in disease. He added that even though disease was no longer considered "irrevocable," it still cost America $35 billion a year.

With history, a booming economy, and elements of the medical community in his corner, President Johnson, the master legislator, pushed his Great Society proposals through Congress in

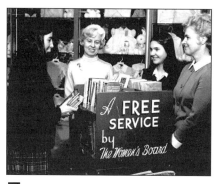

Carol Audet, student, Sacred Heart Academy; Mrs. Stanley Gower, guest speaker; Jacqueline Turgeon, student, Sacred Heart Academy; and Mrs. George Bero, guest speaker help to distribute books to patients.

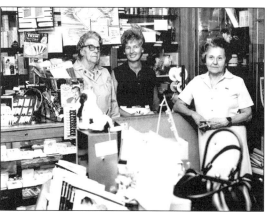

Union Hospital Auxiliary Gift Shop, circa 1970s

proposals through Congress in 1965, and a new era was born. It spawned a predictable "New Deal Redux" of agency acronyms and bureaucratic rules and regulations. Soon, RMPs, CHPs, DONs, and PSROs began to punctuate the conversations of health professionals, flitting about like fledgling sparrows and frequently bumping into one another.

In the meantime, hospitals began forming committees, holding meetings, and hiring additional staff to satisfy administrative

requirements and handle the mounting paperwork. Some considered the extra workload a Faustian pact, while others viewed it as the price one paid for progress. Early patients strenuously objected to having to pay physicians first, then collect from Medicare, which posed a financial hardship. Then hospitals railed against the slow processing of claims, which sometimes made it necessary to borrow money to pay bills. Clearly, some fine-tuning was in order. But regardless of the inconvenience, Medicare and Medicaid were here, and they were not going to go away.

Adding to the headaches was the fact that physicians could now be sued. In a more benign era, when the "good doctor" image prevailed, physicians were exempt from lawsuits under the proviso of "charitable immunity"— but no more. The Darling vs. Charleston Hospital case in 1963 put an end to all that. A young man whose leg had to be amputated because a restrictive cast had cut off blood circulation sued the hospital and won $1 million. It was an unheard-of settlement, but not for long.  The court declared that as an outside industry, governing boards and CEOs would hereafter assume ultimate responsibility for everything the hospital did, including clinical activity of physicians and all others within the hospital's jurisdiction. The court declared that henceforth, physicians and all others would be accountable to the leadership of the hospital. A new industry had been born.

From a humanitarian point of view, the impact of Medicare was immediate and positive, both for elderly patients and health-care professionals. Almost overnight senior citizens rose from "free" patients with fixed incomes to private patients with access to the best medical care available. For the first time, the medical community was receiving adequate reimbursement from a whole segment of the population. It reduced the anxiety of treatment-versus-cost dilemmas for both doctors and patients. At Fall River's Union Hospital, for example, ninety Medicare patients a day were recorded from July 1 to December 31, 1966, the first year the program was in place. There also was a noticeable increase in X-ray patients. And the length of patient stays was already being studied by a utilization committee developed by Sidney W. Rosen, M.D.

Union administration and board members had obviously anticipated the impact of Medicare well in advance and acted accordingly. That year a seven-bed intensive-care unit was built on Stevens 2 West, previously the "men's ward." The Jacob Ziskind laboratory received an addition to house departments of bacteriology, serology, tissue, and chemistry. In addition the X-ray department was overhauled and the blood bank enlarged. At Truesdale, hospital officials also were gearing up. In 1966 they opened the first coronary intensive-care unit in the Fall River area.

# Changing of the Guard

$\mathscr{I}$n 1965 two events occurred that, in retrospect, were to have a profound effect on Union Hospital. One was the passage of Medicare and Medicaid, and the other was the arrival of Frederic "Rick" C. Dreyer, Jr., a thirty-one-year-old graduate of Suffolk University and holder of an M.B.A. from The George Washington University. When Dreyer came on the scene, L.V. Ragsdale, M.D. was administrator and George M. Jackson was his assistant and treasurer. Both men represented the Union Hospital's traditional steady-as-she-goes leadership, which had produced a durable institution boasting three hundred beds and a workforce of nearly a thousand.

Union Hospital administrators traditionally had been local products or longtime area residents. Ragsdale was an exception, a native Alabaman who came to Union in 1955 from Butterworth Hospital in Grand Rapids, Michigan, where he had been medical director. His clinical residency was at Massachusetts General Hospital. Later he became a member of the faculty at the University of Alabama Medical School. Jackson attended The George Washington University and for a time became involved in the tire-and-rubber retail industry. In 1938 he joined Union as treasurer and worked his way up through the ranks. Jackson knew the hospital, the board, and the community. His expertise was in finance. He had been through a depression and a world war. In the break-even world of nonprofit hospitals, as they were then constituted, he was a seasoned manager. And seasoning was highly valued. This was nowhere more evident than on the hospital

board, where trustees served for decades.

Dreyer, conversely, came from an academically oriented postwar generation steeped in advanced organization and management techniques. He was by inclination aggressive and by training sensitive to the need to operate the business side of the enterprise. He had, as he recalls, "a strong sense of the mission to serve others." A wiry and energetic young man full of plans, Dreyer was a devotee of Ray E. Brown, an economist and medical futurist who had the ear of medical leaders and legislators across the nation. Brown, who founded the Duke

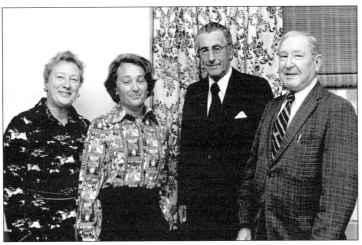

*Mrs. Dorothy Stafford, president of the Women's Board; Mrs. Beverly Udis, past president and chairman of the gift shop; Charles M. Moran, president, Board of Trustees; and George M. Jackson, administrator and treasurer, Union Hospital*

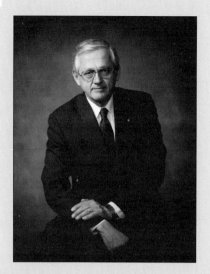

## Frederic C., Dreyer, Jr.

To hear him tell it, Frederic C. "Rick" Dreyer, Jr. might never have gone to college—let alone become chief executive officer of a major hospital system—had it not been for the U.S. Army.

It was in the mid-1950s that Dreyer, high-school dropout, volunteered for the draft and was reassigned from the 101st Airborn Division to the U.S. Army Medical Corps at Fort Sam Houston, Texas. "When they distributed texts entitled *Anatomy* and *Physiology*," he recalls, "I wasn't sure what the words meant but studied the material intensely because I found it so interesting and because I wanted to do anything possible to continue in the program."

Dreyer was later assigned to the 98th General Hospital in Germany, the Seventh Army's center for orthopedic and neurologic services. He began his military experience as a private, and eventually concluded reserve status as a commissioned officer with the rank of major. The adrenaline rush of activity, as trains and helicopters ferried in injured personnel around the clock, lit a fire under Dreyer. "I worked night and day, even volunteering for double

shifts," he says. "It was a fabulous experience. It gave me my first experience with hospital operations. I pursued every possible opportunity to learn and become involved. The military experience led to my career. I was excited about the fascinating world of hospitals and exploded with enthusiasm about becoming involved in any way I might make a difference."

Dreyer, who was trained and certified as an early vintage "EMT," found that he was drawn to the administrative rather than clinical side of medicine. After his discharge, he attended prep school at night and eventually evening-division studies at Saint Joseph's College, Philadelphia. He went on to earn business administration degrees at Worcester's Becker Junior College and Boston's Suffolk University. Subsequently, Dreyer earned a master's degree in business-administration, with a concentration in health-care administration, at The George Washington University, Washington, D.C., and served his administrative residency at Mac-Neal Memorial Hospital in Berwyn, Illinois. In 1965 he came to Union Hospital as an assistant administrator.

In 1969, at age thirty-four Dreyer became the youngest CEO in New England (and perhaps the nation), when he succeeded George M. Jackson as administrator and set out to totally modernize Union's organizational structure and its planning and budgetary process. More than anyone else, he prepared Union for the onslaught of government rules and regulations that followed in the wake of Medicare-Medicaid legislation. In addition, he was a leader in a long campaign for the consolidation of Union and Truesdale hospitals, which was consummated in 1975. And he

played a key role, with the Rev. Dr. Robert P. Lawrence, of First Congregational Church, and others in rekindling a relationship with the Charlton family. The result was a $1 million pledge to the Atwood building fund with many more millions to follow.

Because of his strong leadership, Dreyer has earned his share of critics. But friends and critics alike agree that he is a visionary. It was Dreyer who alerted his colleagues at Charlton to coming trends in American medicine, such as increasing outpatient care, shrinking inpatient services and the rise of prepaid medical services. And it was Dreyer who espoused the regional health concept long before the Southcoast merger took place. Although he retired from Charlton in 1996, he remains active in several organizations and currently is serving a four-year term as a member of the American Hospital Association's Committee on Governance.

In 1996 he received the coveted "Outstanding Citizen Award" by the Greater Fall River Chamber of Commerce and Industry. Also, in 1996 the Southcoast board of trustees, on the recommendation of the auxiliary, named the main lobby at the Charlton site the Frederic C. Dreyer, Jr., lobby. In 1997 the University of Massachusetts/Dartmouth awarded him a doctor of business administration degree (hon.). ◼

University program in health-care administration, had a gift for evaluating trends and forecasting precisely where organized medicine was headed. He was an early advocate of prepayment local and regional arrangements which have evolved into today's HMOs and similar forms of care.

After serving his administrative residency at MacNeal Memorial Hospital in Berwyn, Illinois, Dreyer had three job options—the Pennsylvania Hospital Association; Mary Fletcher Hospital in Burlington, Vermont; and Union Hospital. Friends advised him not to choose Fall River, which was economically flat and losing its young people. The odds were, they told him, that he would not be happy. But Dreyer had a good feeling about the city and its hardworking people who lived in houses overlooking the Taunton River. It was a good place to raise a family.

Although the aging Union leadership heightened the possibility of career advancement, it also was true that these dedicated men offered Dreyer friendship and wisdom as well. And there was another bonus—Dreyer had discovered a "handful" of younger Fall River men who, like himself, wanted to seize the future. In the end he chose Union Hospital simply because it offered him an opportunity to "make an impact." His salary as assistant administrator: $6,500 a year. "I originally planned to stay two or three years at Union," he recalls, "but felt needed here."

One year slipped into another. George M. Jackson became administrator, and in 1968 plans were drawn for an extended-care facility in response to expanding Medicare rolls. The new building would be four stories high and house sixty-four beds for post-acute patients. "Extended care" was a new concept. There was only one other ECF in the country being planned at the time. It was an idea yet to be understood and developed elsewhere across the nation. It would be accompanied by a separate two-story power plant and extend west from the Brayton Building. Union's bed capacity would increase to 370. Employees, too, were on a roll. That year they were given full Blue Cross coverage, a noncontributory pension plan, and increased vacation and sick leave.

Away from work, in the year of the Tet Offensive, there were other things for which to be thankful. The November-December issue of *Pride*, the hospital

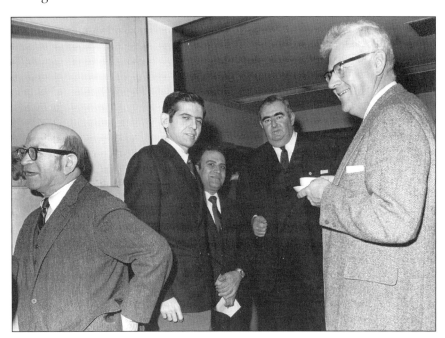

*Samuel Brown, MD; Harvey Reback, MD; Charles Sasson, MD; Thomas Higgins, MD; and Norman Hill, MD*

newsletter, mentioned that Rose Travist and Murial Mosher were happy to welcome their sons home from Vietnam. They were undoubtedly even happier than Evelyn Lavoie, whose vacation in Germany and Austria reportedly left her "completely enchanted" with the Bavarian Alps.

There were sad moments in 1968. One of Union Hospital's most distinguished physicians, John C. Corrigan, died. A noted cardiologist, he was a former president of Union Hospital's medical staff, chief of medicine and the director of medical education. He was commonly referred to as "the physician's physician." Corrigan had the unique honor of having been named a Knight of Saint Gregory by Pope John XXIII. Eugene J. Dionne, chief of the department of dentistry and father of future *Washington Post* columnist

E. J. Dionne, also died that year. Dionne was a generous man who had long run a free dental clinic out of the hospital for needy children and adults.

By now any thoughts Rick Dreyer had entertained about leaving had dissipated. He had been absorbed by the Union "family." In 1969 George M. Jackson resigned as administrator/CEO, and Dreyer succeeded him. He was thirty-four years old and felt, as he recalls, "like a young king who had been handed the crown." His royal exuberance was tempered, however, by the realization that changes were overdue and there was work to be done. Dreyer perceived that Union Hospital's organizational structure would not be sufficient to maintain the status quo, let alone sustain a program of growth, in the government-intensive years to come.

"We are witnessing," he reported in 1969's January-February issue of *Pride*, "changing patterns of physician activity, an increased demand for more hospital services, an intensification

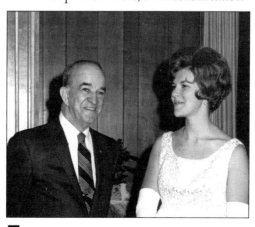

■ *Manual "Manny" Carvalho with Karen S. Dreyer. Mr. Carvalho was a chief engineer at Union Hospital for forty years.*

of educational inservice training activities, a rapidly changing technology, and the ever-increasing participation by government in providing and planning for health services." Peering even further into the future, Dreyer ventured: "Regional health-care planning has already attained enough momentum to be called a movement."

At the top of Dreyer's to-do list was the installation of a budget that would not only modernize business procedures but change the organizational culture of Union Hospital as well. It would represent a quantum leap from the paternalism of the past to a participatory structure, giving department heads more involvement, responsibility, and accountability. It would not be universally popular at first. The absence of a budgeting process and cost-accounting system was common among most hospitals at that time.

In times past, few nonprofit hospitals had budgets per se. Instead they determined what would be spent by what was coming in. It was crucial for administrators to keep close track of what third-party payers, such as Blue Cross, were paying for services. One period, for example, Blue Cross might pay more for emergency room visits—based on customer demand—and another month, certain laboratory tests. If a service was being marginally reimbursed, it made sense not to hike costs. George Jackson, Dreyer recalls, was a juggler nonpareil when it came to keeping such fiscal balls in the air.

"I can remember him coming home from meetings where he had learned, perhaps, that Blue Cross was paying more for a certain service. He'd say, 'I'm going to recommend to the board at the next meeting to raise room rates, effective the first of next month.' Or, he might say, 'I think we should put a dollar on each of the X-ray tests.' That's how he did it, and he could generate $100,000 overnight." Charlton controller William A. Neilan says the system applied to hospital expenditures as well. "The question wasn't, 'Can we afford it?' but rather, 'Is it reimbursable by a third party?'" Later, as limits were imposed, payers and hospitals began devising Byzantine formulas to calculate payments and charges. None, according to Neilan, reflected reality.

Dreyer remembers Jackson scribbling projections on the back of an envelope and reporting revenue levels to the board and what he expected to happen as a result of a new decision by Blue Cross. That was the budget, and the board would applaud. "The philosophy was that the hospital should not generate a profit," Dreyer said. "The board's directive was to come as close to breaking even as possible—that was your fiduciary responsibility. But when we were able to clear a couple hundred thousand a year, the board was happy. Over the years we rarely generated negative financial year end results. Today, under managed care, the financial incentives have changed. Government influences and control have relaxed considerably and

hospitals are encouraged to compete and generate profits—the bigger the better."

Using this tried-and-true conservative approach, Union Hospital stayed clear of most debt and paid off its mortgages. By the same token, there was a distinct possibility that such seat-of-the-pants navigating would run into a thicket as the mingled roles of government and medicine became increasingly complex. Moreover, the fact that all fiscal matters were vested by the board in the administrator meant that under such a centrally controlled system hospital department heads had little notion about what was happening. They depended entirely on approval of the administrator to hire new personnel, initiate pay raises, purchase supplies, and the like. This dependency limited their effectiveness as a resource in solving problems and the ability of the administration to focus on strategic direction and other board issues.

The new budget, Dreyer stressed, would be "decentralized." That is, department managers would be responsible for their own turfs and budgets, planning, and overall operation of their assigned areas. Although ultimately accountable to him, they would make the decisions and act within the scope of predetermined goals and authority in their own backyards. No longer would they be expected to merely react—it was expected that they would press forward with greater individual initiative. "It was highly successful," says Dreyer. "What

happened was more than a delegation exercise. It was truly giving people the sense of ownership, of being responsible, and it worked exceedingly well for years. Today's management theorists and practitioners call this 'empowering employees.' We didn't use that term back then, but employees were being empowered to identify and do things to make the organization progressive, compassionate, caring, and efficient in its service to the community." A few people found the transformation uncomfortable and left. But most employees grew to accept, even embrace, the concept as its benefits became apparent.

Dreyer reinforced the new structure by meeting frequently with department managers and calling in outside experts to monitor the process. He wanted all employees to understand and be part of the planning and budgeting process, to absorb the eternal verity that it was never-ending. He reassured them his door would always be open and that he would be available at any time of the day or night, seven days a week. It was not a cosmetic ploy. For thirty years he met regularly with employees, physicians, volunteers and others. He attended weddings, funerals and caused Charlton to behave like an extended family. Over the course of his career, Dreyer could often be seen walking the halls of the hospital late at night.

# Rules, Rules, and More Rules

There is no better example at a local level of the government's emerging role in medicine than that of utilization review committees (URCs), which were established to provide accountability of hospitals across the nation in the wake of Medicare legislation. Although hospital committees dealt exclusively with Medicare patients at first, Blue Cross eventually adopted the regulations, too. The climate that led to the creation of URCs included:

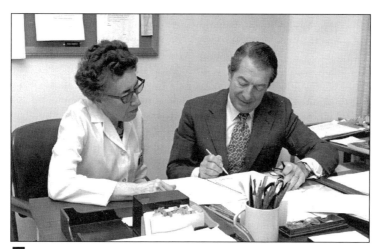

Sidney W. Rosen, MD, utilization review chairman with utilization secretary, Helen Chidsey, late 1960s

- the potential for inflating fees, treatment, and hospital stays
- rising hospital costs that, since World War II, had consistently exceeded the general price index
- rising physician and surgeon fees
- the expanding rolls of Medicare patients

Physicians themselves were pressured by elderly patients and their families to admit them to the hospital, often unnecessarily, or to keep them there longer than needed. In many cases it was a matter of economics for the patients, who paid less for hospitalization than for home care. To assure equity and prevent abuses, URCs were established.

Following preliminary efforts by Dr. Rupert von Trapp in 1966, Dr. Sidney Rosen was appointed to organize and direct the utilization review committee at Union Hospital. Rosen, a board-certified internist, fellow of the American College of Physicians, and fellow of the American College of Gastroenterology, set up a review board that included physicians and administrators. As his task deepened, he turned for assistance to people such as registered nurse Barbara Pietraszek and executive secretary Helen Chidsey. Pietraszek became the only URC nurse coordinator in Massachusetts.

The official goal of the URC was to "conduct a continuing program of review and evaluation of hospital care ... to review the charts of all hospital patients to determine the necessity of services being rendered and the quality of care." If a patient was required to stay in the hospital twelve days or longer, the attending physician had to certify the reason and follow up with frequent reviews. The patient also had to be recertified for the eighteenth and forty-eighth (later changed to thirtieth) days.

In time the URC also assumed the mantle of educator. Through meetings and newsletters, it kept physicians posted about government rules and regulations. Another URC byproduct was statistical studies providing data on subjects such as the length of patient stays and frequency of myocardial infarctions. In a sense, URCs and similar Medicare spinoffs created new disciplines, not to mention soaring sales in the office-supply industry. For example, in a succinct and understated message from the trenches, Chidsey observed, "Patient records alone have become voluminous."

There was more to it than that, of course. The utilization review committee was only the tip of the iceberg. Government agencies associated with health care abounded by the early 1970s, and hospitals had to move quickly to keep up with their game plans. On the up side, President Gerald Ford signed the National Health Planning and Resources Development Act in 1975, which swept away some of the clutter by transferring functions of the Regional Medical Program, Comprehensive Health Planning Act, and venerable Hill-Burton to the newly created regional Health Systems Agencies.

The Health Planning and Resources Development Act decreed that the majority membership of each HSA be composed of consumers, an important step toward the democratization of health planning. Accordingly, Union and Truesdale hospitals began to slate neighborhood meetings as part of their planning agendas. Pecking order—for a building project, for example—now required the hospital to get approval first from neighborhood agencies, then the HSA, before securing a determination of need legislation permit from the State Department of Public Health. Joseph Feitelberg chaired this neighborhood planning agency during the formative years, and Richard Valcourt led this planning initiative for several years thereafter. Clement J. Dowling chaired the regional HSA board. "Clem" Dowling was also a dedicated Charlton trustee for many years. Henry Ashworth of Fall River later chaired the regional HSA.

The subtext of all this federal activity, insofar as hospitals were concerned, was this: plan ahead. That included justifying projects and forecasting their costs to federal agencies, something that had never been done before. As a result of tightening federal controls, hospitals were forfeiting traditional autonomy while gaining revenue. They were becoming increasingly standardized on a nationwide basis. The key to staying ahead of the curve, obviously, was to run faster. In a book of the time called *Five Patients*, writer Michael Crichton (who later penned *Jurassic Park*) summed up modern medicine in a single paragraph:

Medicine has become not a changed profession but a perpetually changing one. There is no longer a sense that one can make a few adjustments and then return to a steady state, for the system will never be stable again.

There is nothing permanent except change itself.

# Through the Looking Glass

*A*s a keen observer of future trends, Rick Dreyer took pains to keep the Union Hospital board of trustees, administration, medical staff, and other employees apprised of changing developments. The idea was not only to inform them but to prepare them for the inevitable changes Union itself would undergo. He accomplished this in part in reports to the board and by writing a regular column called "Comment" in the Union in-house publication, *Pride*.

In 1972 Dreyer was particularly vocal regarding a number of medical trends. There

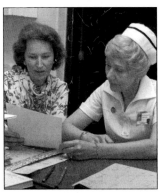

■ *Shirley K. Stretch reviews an application with Virginia Blackburn, RN, employee health nurse. Ms. Stretch was the first director of personnel, later director of human resources. "Shirley knew everyone and reinforced Charlton's sense of caring. She helped me to know what was happening in the lives of the people of Charlton and the community. Her conflict resolving capabilities had a profound impact on the post-merger period," said Rick Dreyer.*

must be a shift, he wrote in one issue, to outpatient care and outreach programs, which were far less expensive than inpatient services and facilities. He recommended that they be used whenever possible. He noted that embryonic "health-care corporations (systems) are being formed, offering contracted prepaid health services." It was futile to resist the external (largely governmental) forces generating such changes, he stated. Better to adapt, to bend the future to one's own advantage. After all, he added, quoting Ray E. Brown, medicine "simply mirrors the transition of our own society."

During this period, it also was Brown who noted a recent tendency of the public to regard the emergency services department as the "gateway to the health-care system." Although their frequent visits were often misdirected, he felt that the phenomenon indicated a public desire for medical care under a centralized system. The independent family doctor was vanishing. The public was ready for a "composite doctor" surrounded by an entire spectrum of medical services.

■ *Cardiac care unit open house, 1966, Lawton S. Brayton; Eleanor E. Presbrey, RN; Charles M. Moran; and Patricia Daley, RN*

Dreyer took this concept a step further: Hospitals "now are assuming a new commitment— providing the framework for keeping all people healthy .... We want this hospital to be the focal point of a health-care system that includes all the people." The gravitational spin of the hospital, it seemed, was picking up speed and pulling ever more concepts, including prevention, into its orbit—rather like, as Brown might have said, a shopping center.

# Digits and Decimals

*I*n 1969 the Union Hospital personnel department consisted of one part-time employee hired to interview job applicants. By 1971 it had expanded to a bona fide department, headed initially by Eleanor Presbrey, R.N., then Shirley K. Stretch, with four other full-time employees. A native of Connecticut, Stretch had a background in banking and newspapers. Her writing

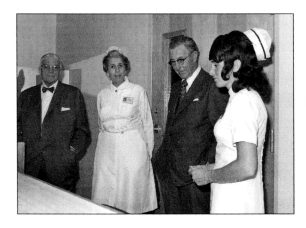

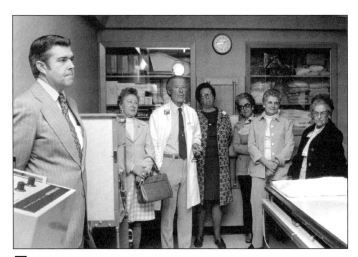

Dedication of the radiology special procedures room, January 1975, George R. Boyce, president of Union Hospital; Mrs. Birtwell Stafford, president of the Women's Board; Eugene A. Field, MD, chief radiologist; Mrs. Joseph Merritt, trustee; Mrs. Thomas Davol, member of the Women's Board; Mrs. David Cohen, member of the Women's Board; Mrs. George M. Jackson, member of the Women's Board

was one of several promising young administrators brought on board by Dreyer. Other notable picks included Edward M. Klaman and Arthur J. Sampson as administrative residents, both of whom eventually became vice presidents responsible for various hospital operations. "We had an affiliation with The George Washington University," Dr. Arthur Anctil recalls, "Rick would bring in the best people. It was a smart move, because he could choose among them."

Anctil, former medical-staff president and board trustee, particularly applauds the hiring of William A. Neilan, a mid-career professional, as controller. Neilan,

experience on a Rhode Island weekly, made her a natural to assume public-relations chores as well. The personnel department not only processed new employees, it administered the wage-and-salary program. It also served as a training and inservice resource for other departments.

Life was getting brisker at Union—perhaps even more officious. It was a hospital with a full plate. That year, for example, the sixty-four-bed Moran Building was completed. Dedicated to Charles M. Moran, the longtime president of the Union Hospital board of trustees, it was accompanied by a separate two story, state-of-the art boiler plant and laundry (later converted to a computer and communications center). Administrative technology was updated, too. Systems analyst Carl O. Weaver developed a closed computer network that freed Union

from having to share a system with other hospitals through the Massachusetts Hospital Association. This innovative move made it possible to process records on site, saving Union money by expediting the paying of bills and keeping better track of late charges.

Such technology might elicit yawns today, but it was a source of amazement twenty-five years ago. A 1973 *Pride* article related that "the computer area is closed off, but one can watch through the large glass windows this wonder of wonders." And later: "They even had their own language—RPG II—computer talk." Even the copy machine provoked gasps. It "not only copies but will reduce any size original to either a legal- or letter-size copy."

Weaver, a graduate of the University of Rhode Island, had joined Union Hospital in 1970 from the home offices of Massachusetts Mutual Insurance Company. He

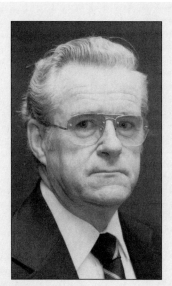

William A. Neilan was controller from 1971 to 1989, and became senior vice president and treasurer in 1990. He is credited with providing financial expertise for the challenging era of Medicare-Medicaid.

who was in the process of being relocated to the Midwest as a result of the closure of the Firestone Rubber & Latex Products Company plant in Fall River, "could take all the accounting jargon and translate it for the medical staff. He had a way of taking bad news and putting a good spin on it." Dreyer saw another dimension: "During eras of government infringement and extraordinary controls, Bill Neilan kept us financially stable when other hospitals were failing." It was a tribute that the thrifty John D. Flint, the "father of Union Hospital," would have appreciated. In the waning months of 1973, a portrait of Flint, the silvery-maned patriarch, was hung in the Trustees Room of the Moran Building.

# Three into One Will Go

*T*he year was 1972, and the last three Fall River Diploma Schools of Nursing were graduating their final classes, ending eighty-seven years of tradition. In one respect, it was a bittersweet experience. On the other hand, it heralded the future. Two years before, the Union, Truesdale, and Saint Anne's schools of nursing had combined to create a new entity the Fall River Diploma School of Nursing. The first classes had begun in September 1970. The merger was not a sudden development; it had been evolving for some time. Nursing was changing, like all of medicine. And community needs were changing as well.

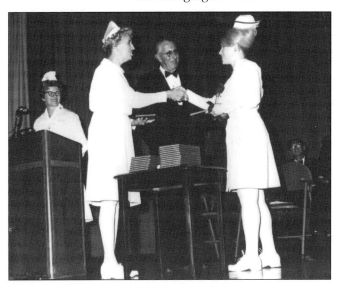

Eleanor E. Presbrey, Union Hospital director of nursing, awards diplomas with the assistance of Charles Moran, board of trustees president. Joyce McGanka, assistant director of the school of nursing stands at podium while George Bounakes, MD and Rev. Dr. Robert P. Lawrence look on, 1968.

Now, as the twenty-six members of the Union Hospital School of Nursing class of 1972 surmounted the Ziskind Auditorium stage, one-by-one, to pick up their diplomas, memories hung in the air. For young graduates such as Kerry Darcy and Zita Ferreira, the memories no doubt centered on the recent past—on classes, instructors, and good times. For older participants, such as director of nursing Eleanor E. Presbrey, they stretched back three generations to a time when nurses toiled on the front lines of social change.

It had been the same at the Truesdale Hospital School of Nursing's last graduation. Founded by Dr. Ralph French in 1912, the school inspired a loyalty all its own. The pastoral beauty of the campus provided a panoramic backdrop to the event. For example, Isabelle S. Ward, a 1925 graduate, still remembers Dr. Frederick R. Barnes parking his car in the same spot every day—a seemingly inconsequential yet tenacious thread to the past. She recalls making rounds in the hospital, the sound of footsteps in the corridors, and time spent with the Providence Public Mission Association going out into the community.

Those early days seem bathed in the special glow of an unjaded world. In 1927 Mary K. Nelson, Truesdale's first nursing supervisor, paid a visit to the campus. Nelson had volunteered for duty in World War I, then stayed on in Europe after the armistice. Now director of the

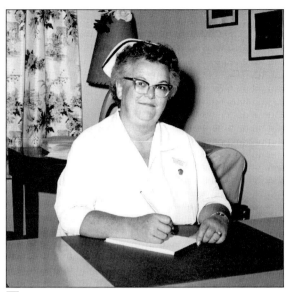

Edna Lambert, RN, instructor and associate director of the school of nursing at Truesdale for nearly twenty years.

American Hospital School of Nursing in Constantinople (Istanbul), she captivated the students with stories of exotic places and customs. Before leaving, she presented the school with a picture of "Nightingale Barracks," the crude structure where Florence Nightingale had ministered to the wounded and dying during the Crimean War.

Sitting in the audience that October evening was Delight S. Jones, R.N., who in 1927 had been appointed director of nursing. A charismatic and dedicated professional, Jones had completely reorganized the nursing department in a drive to upgrade patient care and nursing-student education. Jones, a graduate of both the Massachusetts Memorial Hospital School of Nursing and Columbia University, had outfitted the basement of the nursing home as a bedside-care classroom, obtained a dissectible model for teaching anatomy and surgery, beefed up the reference library, and added nurse helpers as a way to eliminate non-educational routine duties. She also imposed an eight-hour schedule and separated obstetrical and pediatric services.

In 1931 the overcrowded Truesdale Hospital School of Nursing had received a boost with the dedication of the Mitchell House, a new nurses' home financed by Ruth Charlton Mitchell. It came just in time for the Great Depression, which would stretch the resources of the nursing profession to the limit. Income would shrink and the number of non-paying patients grow. In 1938 the annual report disclosed that the size of the nursing school and number of graduate nurses had increased "due to a higher daily average number of patients." World War II and a thriving postwar economy ended this hand-to-mouth existence. Having survived the crucible, the Truesdale Hospital School of Nursing, like its Union Hospital counterpart, continued to serve the community in a selfless and progressive spirit.

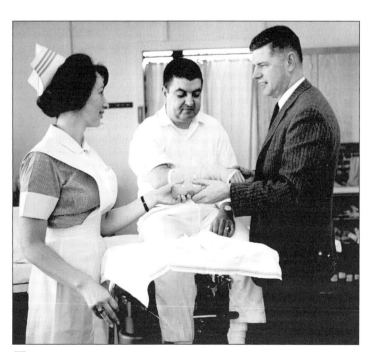

Bruce Derbyshire, MD, demonstrates bandage wrapping for a student nurse on orderly Eddie Amaral, Truesdale Hospital.

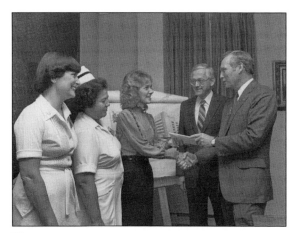

Judy McCann, vice president; Mary Ann Wordell; and Barbara Sporleder of the Truesdale Hospital Nurses Alumnae Association present a donation to Union-Truesdale Hospital Chairman Donald H. Ramsbottom and CEO Frederic C. Dreyer, Jr.

According to Class of 1940 graduate, Dorothy Winter, the program which began with four students enrolled in a three-year diploma program, graduated 923 students, many of whom served or are serving in positions of responsibility around the world.

The story of the Union Hospital School of Nursing had begun in 1885 with the establishment of the Fall River Hospital and its nursing school. With the merger in 1900 of all three medical facilities, the first Union School of Nursing class was formed.

In those early years, the nursing corps played a particularly crucial role in the advancement of medicine in Fall River—a teeming textile giant swarming with immigrants, appalling social conditions, and disease. In addition to their hospital roles, nurses visited homes in the role of health advisers, helped deliver babies, and made sure impoverished children were properly nourished. They showed poor families how to get the most from their meager incomes by providing a healthy environment and good food. And they even sponsored English instruction for those who wanted to learn.

Nurses did the unglamorous but vital "grunt" work that abounds in all medical facilities. And doctors depended on them to keep things running. They put in long hours and took pride in their work. They were there for Fall River's citizens during wars, epidemics, and hard times. And they often were leaders. In the early days, nurses routinely served as administrators. In 1942 Jennie Smithies, R.N., Union Hospital School of Nursing graduate, was appointed hospital superintendent. Smithies, a colorful, take-charge type, became something of a legend in Fall River.

The Union Hospital School of Nursing instilled in its students a reverence for excellence and compassion. It was known for the

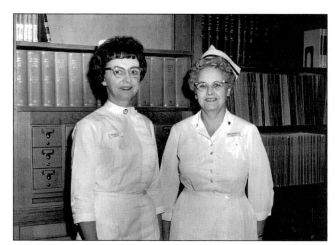

Supervisors Barbara Arnold and Emily Bellman of Truesdale Hospital

academic rigor of its programs. In 1913, for example, the curriculum was lengthened to three years in response to steadily advancing medical knowledge. A year later, physical therapy—an especially vital discipline in industrial Fall River—was added to its course work. In 1922 the nursing school library was expanded. And in 1933 Elizabeth House, a nurses' home, was built using funds expressly provided by the late philanthropist Elizabeth Stevens.

After World War II, the emphasis in nursing education slowly but inexorably began to shift to centers of higher education. Nursing had long since left its bandage-and-aspirin days. It was becoming, as everything else in medicine, highly technical. It required more education with better equipment and laboratories. Nursing schools were getting to be expensive propositions. Universities and colleges, on the other hand, with their swelling popularity and wealth, were tailor-made to meet these demands.

In Fall River, as elsewhere, nurses remained in great demand, and it eventually became a practical matter to establish nursing programs in institutions such as Bristol Community College (BCC) and, thereafter, Southeast Massachusetts University (SMU). But until graduating classes could begin rolling off the line, the Fall River Diploma School of Nursing served as a bridge from the outgoing hospital schools to institutions of higher learning. It

provided an abundant supply of nurses to Fall River hospitals during a time of national shortage. When BCC, SMU and other institutions were able to take up the slack, the Fall River Diploma School of Nursing, as planned, was dissolved.

In the meantime, nursing students had changed since the 1950s. They were more independent and less accepting of the social-support roles previously assigned to their mothers.

In a 1972 interview, Eleanor Presbrey addressed this phenomenon, saying, "This generation is the most mobile that

the United States has ever seen.... The young all want to do their 'thing,' although to most of the older generation they all seem to conform to their own standards even more than our generation.... The rugged individualist is fast disappearing." Postwar affluence, Presbrey added, also had a decided effect. "You try harder when you're hungry," she said.

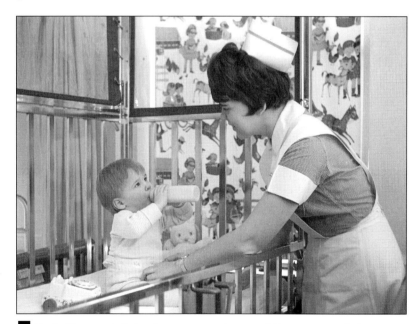

*Beth (Lawson) Schuchman cares for a toddler at Truesdale Hospital, circa 1968.*

# Raise High the Roofbeam

*O*n December 7, 1971, the Charles M. Moran Building was dedicated at Union Hospital. It was an unusual date, to be sure. But as Rabbi Moshe Babin, pastor of Temple Beth-El, pointed out in the invocation, the irony was appropriate. On the anniversary of Pearl Harbor, an attack that had killed nearly two thousand Americans, he reminded listeners that on this occasion Fall River was rededicating itself to the "preservation and improvement of human life."

Guests that winter day gathered in the Moran Building's new lobby—still smelling of fresh paint in soft shades of blue, green, and yellow—then adjourned to a large room on the first floor for the dedication. Speakers lauded Charles M. Moran for his more than twenty-five years on the board of trustees, where he served as president of the board and of the corporation. As chairman of the building committee, he had had a leading role in the construction of the sixty-bed Brayton Building, completed in 1959. During Moran's watch, the Union complex had grown from two major buildings into a complex of seven.

Among those present at the dedication were Moran; retired administrator George Jackson; Dr. Daniel Rubenstein, retired director of the Massachusetts Division of Hospital Facilities; state senator Mary Fonseca; architect William Riley; contractor Frank L. Collins;

George J. Bounakes, M.D., president of the Union Hospital medical staff; and Union Hospital administrator/CEO Frederic C. Dreyer, Jr.

The Moran Building—a sixty-four bed, thirty-two room medical and surgical facility—originally had been planned as an extended-care facility (ECF) to handle the growing number of Medicare patients. At the time there was only one forty-bed, approved ECF in the greater Fall River area. The new facility would house recovering patients who still needed a hospital environment. It would offer, among other features, a paramedic station, physical therapy, rehabilitative nursing care, and restorative services. The object was to provide a bridge between regular inpatient care and discharge to the home or other medical facilities. In the eleventh hour of construction, a bureaucratic snaggle involving Medicare reimbursement procedures forced the facility to undergo a costly conversion to acute care. State-of-the art medical and surgical intensive-care units

were constructed in areas designed as large recreational areas for ECF patients.

The Moran Building was contiguous to the main hospital, providing easy access to medical staff and service areas. It consisted of four floors and was connected to the west wing of the Brayton Building. That same year, a new two-story state-of-the-art boiler plant also was completed at Union Hospital. The first floor housed a gas-fed incinerator with "air scrubbers" to satisfy emerging environmental requirements.

It was connected by tunnel to the rest of the hospital at the south wing of the Brayton Building and the "old laundry," which some years earlier had been converted to workshops. But even as the guests mingled at the dedication, plans were afoot for a total health-care facility and a physicians' office building, which would be connected to the west of the Moran Building.

The plan was to relocate seventy physicians (in time, even more) from their various scattered

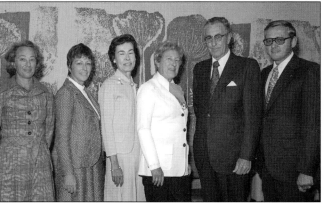

*Dedication day at the Moran Building, 1972, Mrs. Sanford (Beverly) Udis, Mrs. Harvey (Sylvia) Reback, Mrs. Robert (Sue) Hutton, Mrs. Birtwell (Dorothy) Stafford, Charles M. Moran and Frederic C. Dreyer, Jr.*

locations to a centralized location connected to the hospital, with the hospital providing clinical and business support services to the physicians. It was to be a hospital-physicians collaboration that would have been twenty years ahead of its time. But it was not to be. A powerful "old guard" segment of the board opposed the proposal. The architectural rendering by Richie Associates of Boston and the organizational plan to bring doctors and hospital together was doomed to be shelved. Rick Dreyer describes this as one of the major disappointments of his career. "The development of this program," Dreyer says, "would likely have changed the history of Fall River hospitals. It would have positioned Union Hospital and its physicians to take initiatives at that time which were consequently not pursued again until the 1990s when national influences under managed care made such a move obvious. The project was financially viable with no regulatory or other serious impediments in the way of accomplishing it.

"It was frustrating," Dreyer concludes, "not to be able to proceed with that project."

A poignant footnote to construction occurred when twenty-four abandoned graves had to be dug up to make room for the Moran Building. It was a delicate situation. Efforts were made to locate heirs of the deceased, but there was not much to go on. Time and the elements had scoured names and dates from the headstones. So many generations had passed that even historical memory was obliterated. Finally, the remains were recovered and placed in a common grave at Oak Grove Cemetery with full services. Rev. Ferdinand Loungeway, who officiated, observed that the quality

and dignity of a civilization is reflected in the way it buries its dead. The removal of the bodies and construction of the new facility both reaffirmed Union Hospital's reverence for the dead and its commitment to the living.

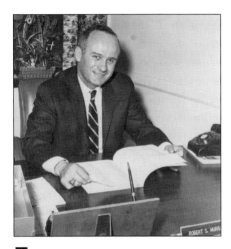

Robert S. Murray, president, Truesdale Hospital

# A Cup of Soup

*F*ormer Truesdale physician David S. Greer remembers that talk about consolidating Union and Truesdale hospitals started in earnest around 1965. Others are not so sure. But it is a fact that thoughts of some kind of consolidation began to percolate in the mid-sixties. New players were beginning to come on the scene in greater numbers. Charles M. Moran and his veteran colleagues were seeing a younger cohort of leadership represented by such people as Truesdale Hospital board president Robert Murray who, like Rick Dreyer, came from a working-class background.

The composition of the medical staffs had changed, too. There was still an aura of exclusivity at Truesdale and matching class resentment at Union, but younger doctors tended to be outsiders without local baggage. Raised amid postwar populism and sharing similar educational backgrounds, many viewed the Union-Truesdale rivalry as slightly sophomoric.

Their lack of interest in perpetuating the rivalry, combined with glaring medical duplication in Fall River and the prospect of government intervention, began to erode the status quo.

In November 1968 Truesdale gingerly crossed the dance floor when Robert Murray met attorney Harold Hudner, president of Saint Anne's Hospital board of trustees, for a cup of soup at the Howard Johnson's restaurant in Swansea. The focus of their conversation was how to develop cooperation among Fall River hospitals for the purpose of "improving health services, eliminating duplication of services,

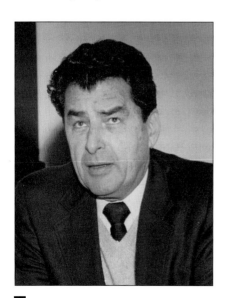

David S. Greer, MD

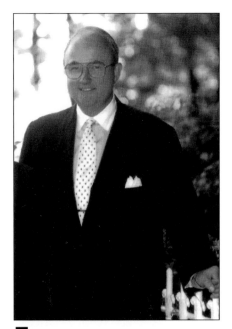

Sumner James Waring, Jr., a
twenty-five-year trustee who
encouraged and influenced
trustees, physicians and the
community at large to embrace
and support the Union-
Truesdale merger

and lowering hospital costs for
patients." Murray recalls Hudner
saying, "You don't think we can do
anything with Charlie Moran, do
you?" Murray replied that, no, he
did not think so. It was common
knowledge that Charles Moran was
no more disposed toward
consolidation than he had been in
the 1950s, when he clashed with
Truesdale's chairman of the board,
John B. Cummings. So Murray and
Hudner ruled Union Hospital out
and focused on the possibilities
between Truesdale and Saint
Anne's.

Following that rendezvous,
selected board members from
Truesdale and Saint Anne's began
meeting periodically at Saint
Anne's cafeteria for informal
brainstorming sessions on how best
to combine services and eliminate
duplication between the two
hospitals. Saint Anne's
representatives included Hudner,
James Waldron, Sister Jean Marie,
and Joseph Feitelberg. Truesdale
fielded Murray, Robert Truesdale
(Philemon's son), and Sumner
James Waring, Jr. In March 1969
board members solicited outside
expertise when they met at White's
restaurant to hear William
Robinson, executive director of the
Massachusetts Hospital
Association, discuss "improving
health services and eliminating
duplication of effort."

Talks were moving along
smoothly when word filtered back
to Union Hospital about the
developing partnership. Officials
there relayed a message through
Dr. Greer that Union would like to
be invited to participate in this
"community endeavor." In the
interest of fairness, Saint Anne's
and Truesdale extended an
invitation, which was promptly
accepted. There followed a five-
year running drama featuring an
ensemble cast of four hospitals,
which would also include Hussey
Hospital, also in Fall River, with the

Paul V. Stevens, trustee,
Charlton Memorial Hospital. As
a trustee for seventeen years,
Mr. Stevens devoted his
immense energy and talent to
promote the success of Charlton
Memorial Hospital and the
construction of the Atwood
Building.

spotlight rarely straying from
Union and Truesdale. Representing
Union were Charles M. Moran,
Henry Ashworth, Paul V. Stevens,
Bertram Yaffe, and Rick Dreyer.

In June 1969 the first meeting
of the newly created Fall River Joint
Committee for Health Services was
held. The mission of the committee,
which was formed with the
inclusion of Union Hospital, was
identical to that of the
Truesdale–Saint Anne's liaison—to
pursue cooperation and end
duplication of services. Throughout
that summer and into the fall, the
committee examined a number of
plans designed to serve the health
needs of the greater Fall River area.
The study led to the presentation of
this motion: "One medical staff
with one health corporation should
evolve for the Fall River area." In
January 1970 Truesdale voted "aye"
but Union and Saint Anne's vetoed
the idea.

The setback was
disappointing. Nevertheless, talks
resumed at a new venue, the
Quequechan Club, where Fall River

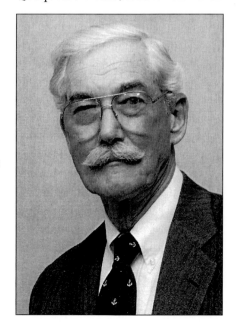

business elites had congregated for more than seventy-five years and consummated deals over plates of scrod and steaming cups of coffee. Perhaps participants hoped that the ghostly presences of John D. Flint and Frank Stevens would sit in on the joint committee and nudge things along.

As it turned out, even the hallowed Quequechan Club and its gallery of departed greats could not soothe consolidation jitters. For example, the joint committee conducted a study to determine the feasibility of consolidating obstetrics and pediatrics at one hospital. The study revealed that Fall River hospitals were operating the services at a deficit of $700,000 per year, which patients had to make up with rate hikes. The data clearly supported consolidation. While members of the committee did not dispute the conclusion, they seemed unable to proceed. "Complications, including a question of consolidation or merger, hindered final action," wrote the joint committee chairman, attorney James T. Waldron in the "Waldron Report."

Amid the indecision, there was a ray of hope. In the course of its investigation, the committee uncovered an urgent need for pediatric intensive- and neonatal-care units in the Fall River area. All three hospital boards of trustees agreed that Saint Anne's should supply these special- care units. The Catholic institution filed its requests through the proper channels and was granted the necessary approvals.

The next step, as the joint committee saw it, was to appoint a subcommittee to explore in depth the advisability of consolidating or merging the three hospitals. The subcommittee was charged with answering the question: Would merger or consolidation of Saint Anne's Hospital, Truesdale Hospital, and Union Hospital substantially improve health care in Fall River? The subcommittee met for the first of thirteen sessions on November 23, 1970. By March it had its answer: yes. The majority of hospital representatives voted agreement. But the unity was short-lived. Agreement was anything but a fait accompli.

In position papers that month, hospital representatives expressed widely divergent opinions about what constituted consolidation. Concept was one

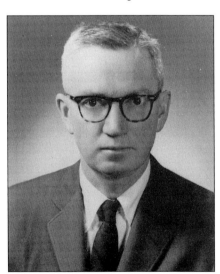

■ *Attorney Philip S. Brayton, chairman, Truesdale Hospital, 1966-1971*

thing, implementation another. The Truesdale paper, prepared by president Robert Murray, board chairman Philip Brayton, and medical-dental staff president Frank Collins, Jr., M.D., pushed for a new hospital at a new site or, barring that, consolidation of services of the three hospitals, with the identities of the institutions being preserved. In the latter scenario, Truesdale suggested boards of trustees should remain intact until attrition reduced their numbers.

Saint Anne's Hudner believed neighborhood health centers should be established under a new corporation set up by the three hospitals. The centers would focus on preventive medicine and conduct tests for measles, tuberculosis, and other common diseases. Hudner recommended that Saint Anne's take over all of the maternity wards in the area, leaving Union to focus on its cancer and stroke clinics, social services, and extended care. In addition, the well-equipped Union facility could do most of the lab work for all three hospitals. Hudner believed Truesdale should be supported in its quest to build a new hospital, where it could specialize in gynecology and diseases such as multiple sclerosis and muscular dystrophy.

Writing on behalf of Union, trustee and subcommittee alternate Henry Ashworth urged consolidation of services at one site. He reminded the joint committee that the supply of qualified doctors, medical support staff, and funds for equipment was limited in Fall River. To complicate matters, duplication and waste was coming under increasing scrutiny by third-party payers, who were "hard-nosed about our costs." Ashworth believed the merger or consolidation of three "or even two" hospitals would forge a greater bargaining chip in attracting outside support from entities such as teaching hospitals in Boston.

A fourth position paper was submitted by George M. Jackson, recently retired Union Hospital administrator. It differed sharply from Ashworth's and was endorsed by Charles M. Moran. According to Jackson,

- Fall River had few problems regarding availability and adequacy of inpatient hospital care and treatment.
- Many area residents were unaware of services offered by local hospitals.
- An expansion of outpatient services was needed, particularly maternal and child-health programs.
- Consolidation of some

hospital services, such as obstetrics, pediatrics, and certain outpatient clinics, would be beneficial.

By now it was clear to Waldron—a tough, suspender-wearing labor lawyer—that the talks had reached an impasse. "For thirty-nine months," he wrote, "the question of improving health care for the people of the Greater Fall River area has been raised and discussed formally and informally among hospital trustees and in committees. In the opinion of the chair, we have not been successful." It was his belief, Waldron added, that merger or consolidation of the three hospitals was "impossible at this time."

Waldron acknowledged that the talks had not been without value. They had stimulated an exchange of ideas and information. Each hospital had shared financial information, as well as data about hospital operations, previously held by each as "privileged information." Moreover, the subcommittee on consolidation had been allowed to visit and examine each institution. That alone was precedent-breaking. Union's board president Charles M. Moran, in fact, turned his visit into an intelligence foray. Noticing that Truesdale's roof was in need of repair, Moran, who owned a roofing company, wondered aloud to a colleague if the hospital might be having financial problems. Later events would prove that Moran, was right.

# Consolidation

In the absence of a consolidation plan by the subcommittee, Waldron submitted his own. Waldron's plan called for Truesdale and Saint Anne's to pursue consolidation of services. Recommendations included

- one medical staff for both hospitals
- preserving hospital names
- establishing a stroke unit at Truesdale, with facilities at Hussey Hospital
- merging obstetrics and pediatrics at Saint Anne's
- eventual consolidation of Truesdale and Saint Anne's properties (one site)
- inclusion of Union Hospital when legal roadblocks involving its trusts and mortgages were cleared.

Waldron noted that while talks had been proceeding, Union Hospital had started construction of the Moran Building and a new power plant. "We who are interested in hospital work in the Greater Fall River area are proud of the accomplishments made by the Union Hospital," he wrote. "We should devote our efforts in bringing to fruition the opening of this extended care facility [Moran Building]." In other words, Union Hospital was a force to be reckoned with.

*I*t was the middle of 1971, and everything was back to square one. After three years, Fall River's hospitals had succeeded in establishing lines of communication but little else. To Robert Murray and his colleagues, it seemed that Union's Charles Moran wanted to absorb Truesdale, not consolidate. "He thought if he waited long enough," Murray recalls, "Truesdale would die from its own weight." Even though Moran stayed in the background during negotiations, Murray believes he was "calling the shots." Absorbing Truesdale was unthinkable. It would obliterate seventy years of history and a national reputation for excellence.

Yet Murray, who had originated talks between the hospitals, knew the clock was running down. Something had to

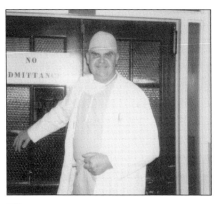

Alan Simpson, MD, Truesdale Hospital

be done. It was his hope that duplication could be eliminated without sacrificing hospital identity—at least for a while. Saint Anne's Hudner concurred. Better to consolidate over time than overnight. Once again Truesdale and Saint Anne's decided to go it alone. Hospital representatives began meeting quietly aboard the battleship *U.S.S. Massachusetts*,

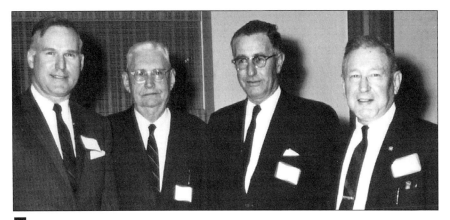

Attorney Francis T. Meagher, trustee; L.V. Ragsdale, MD, medical director and administrator; Charles M. Moran, board president; and George M. Jackson, treasurer attend a Christmas party in the Brayton Building, 1965.

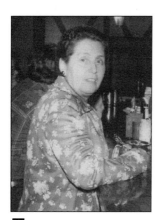

Hazel Davis, RN, head nurse, Union Hospital, circa 1970s

moored in Fall River's Battleship Cove. A wardroom once privy to speculation about war strategy now resonated with talk about other matters.

On October 30, 1971, *The Fall River Herald News* ran a sixty-point banner headline across its front page: "St. Anne's, Truesdale Hospitals to Merge." The dam had broken, and two Fall River institutions—one religious, the other secular—had finally come together. The article began,

Saint Anne's Hospital and Truesdale Hospital will merge into a single corporation. Each will become a unit of the proposed Greater Fall River Medical Center, Inc. The target date for accomplishment of the merger is Jan. 1, 1972. Should delay ensue, an ultimate date of June 30, 1972 has been set.

Here was the fait accompli, the "done deal." It was, as the newspaper reported, "the culmination of discussions which began in November, 1968." All that remained were handshakes and a few strokes of a pen.

The agreement hammered out between Saint Anne's and Truesdale echoed the consolidation plan devised by Waldron—most notably, the formation of one medical staff and board of trustees, transfer of obstetrics and pediatrics to Saint Anne's, and retention of hospital identities (called Truesdale Unit and Saint Anne's Unit). It neutralized the explosive issue of abortion by banning birth control and abortion procedures at Saint Anne's. Neither doctors nor support medical personnel were required to perform or take part in operations that contradicted religious or moral beliefs. Moreover, most doctors could "more or less" restrict their practice to one of the hospitals, which kept alive a cherished Truesdale tradition. As for Union Hospital, it was invited to join the consolidation once it was free of legal entanglements.

In the meantime, Waldron recommended establishing a nonprofit "human service corporation" (HSC) that would develop total health services for the greater Fall River area. "We must remove ourselves from being just the guardians of bricks and mortar and recognize our trusteeship as a public trust for every man," he wrote. The HSC presumably would be above parochialism. Its board of trustees would be composed of representatives from all three

hospitals, the city of Fall River, and the nursing-home industry. It would be managed by a full-time coordinator skilled at obtaining state and federal grants, which would be needed to sustain HSC programs.

In effect the human-service corporation would fine-tune the balancing act of services among Union, Saint Anne's, and Truesdale hospitals. It would provide a nip here and a tuck there while tentatively exploring the benefits of centralized laundry facilities or—more boldly—computer services. Like Hudner's position paper, the HSC voiced support for neighborhood clinics "where needed." With the proposed HSC running interference, Truesdale and Saint Anne's continued their end-sweep toward consolidation.

As it turned out, the players never crossed the goal line. The January 1 date for consolidation came and went. Saint Anne's was having a crisis of conscience. Would consolidation with a secular institution subvert canonical law? Would Saint Anne's be morally liable even though birth control and abortion were restricted to the Truesdale site? What would happen when, as planned, the hospitals consolidated their real estate? Misgivings deepened. Finally, Saint Anne's pulled out. On June 22, 1972, *The Fall River Herald News* ran another front-page story reporting that the merger was dead. Saint Anne's statement was blunt.

An outright merger with Truesdale Hospital or any nonsectarian institution would result in St. Anne's

Hospital's loss of its identity as a Catholic institution and the impossibility to adhere to the ethical and moral directives of the Catholic Church. We wish, however, to remain fully involved in the planning of comprehensive health care for the Fall River area.

Years later, Charlton Memorial Hospital, led by Donald Ramsbottom and Rick Dreyer, also would attempt to consolidate with Saint Anne's. Negotiations would be extensive and in-depth. In the end, Saint Anne's would again withdraw for religious reasons. Meanwhile, Truesdale leaders expressed keen "disappointment" while putting on a conciliatory face. What could be done in the face of such conviction? And yet, as Robert Murray discovered, the game was not over yet. Truesdale physician

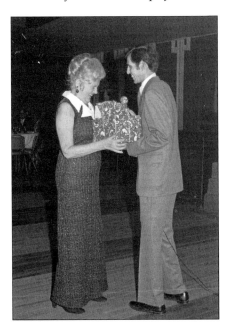

*Theresa Sullivan, RN, night supervisor and Harvey Reback, MD, president of the medical staff at Union, later chief of medicine of Charlton Memorial, at the annual Christmas party*

David Greer was about to call in a play from the sidelines. Greer, a community activist and future Nobel laureate who served as unpaid chief of medicine at Earl E. Hussey Hospital, suggested to Murray a concept that rapidly evolved into a new lease on life.

Under the concept, Truesdale would merge with Hussey and purchase land on the city-owned Hussey site for the construction of a 220-bed hospital, to be called the Fall River Health and Human Services Center, Inc. Health services and medical staffs would be combined, and ambulatory services would be increased. The District Nursing Association, Hussey Rehabilitation Center, and Cerebral Palsy Rehabilitation Center would be centralized at the new hospital. In addition, affiliations with universities and other health-related educational institutions would be strengthened. On November 8, 1972, the *Fall River Herald News* published details of the plan, including the fact that approval of the city council would be required.

As Murray recalls, Rick Dreyer and Union Hospital "came out with guns blazing." According to Union Hospital leaders, the newspaper article was the first they had heard about "the concept," as it was called. In a letter to Dr. Ann H. Pettigrew, acting director of the Division of Medical Care

of the state Department of Public Health, Dreyer lambasted "the concept," saying it would result in "one of the most costly and embarrassing mistakes of the century in Fall River."

That was not just Dreyer's personal opinion; he was speaking on behalf of the Union Hospital Planning Committee, which included Charles M. Moran, George R. Boyce, George M. Jackson, and Paul V. Stevens plus physicians Arthur K. Smith, Thomas Higgins, Daniel L. Mooney, and Sydney W. Rosen. The committee was unanimous in its conclusion that the Truesdale-Hussey plan was bloated with duplication and unnecessary expense. Dreyer petitioned Clement J. Dowling, president of the board of directors of Region VII Comprehensive Health Planning, Inc., to allow Union Hospital to present its own long-range plan "as soon as possible."

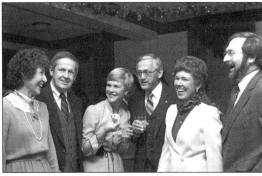

*Dr. and Mrs. Francis M. James, past president of medical staff and trustee; Mr. and Mrs. Frederic C. Dreyer, Jr., president and CEO; and Dr. and Mrs. Ronald A. Schwartz, chief of medicine and trustee at the auxiliary holiday party at New Bedford Country Club.*

In the January 1973 *Pride* newsletter, Dreyer wrote that Union's long-range plan was virtually identical "in concept" to that of Truesdale-Hussey, except Union favored development at an existing site—its own. After all, he reasoned, Union was listed among the top twenty Massachusetts hospitals. It was one of the largest and most up-to-date institutions in the region. Union already had most of what was needed to fulfill the plan and could do it at less than a third of what it would cost to build a new hospital. For example, Truesdale's acute-care service could be transferred to Union, which had available space, while chronic- and long-term-care services could be channeled to Truesdale without the expense of new construction. In short, the citizens of greater Fall River would benefit from better and more economical use of medical care facilities and services already in place.

Despite Union Hospital's opposition, the Fall River city council voted in favor of the Truesdale-Hussey proposal early in 1973. Negotiations proceeded, and the Fall River Medical and Human Services Center, Inc., shortly came into being. In March Ruth Hurley, chairperson of Hussey Hospital, extended an invitation to Union Hospital to join. Criteria for joining included the "transfer of title to all property and assets of the Union Hospital in Fall River." The deadline for acceptance was March 31, a scant eleven days later. Dreyer responded in a position paper that such a transfer was impossible without the approval of the hospital corporation, which, under hospital bylaws, would not be able to arrange a vote before the deadline. Even then, extensive legal studies would need to precede such a vote.

Dreyer did not stop there but proceeded to point out what he perceived to be other flaws in the center's proposal. Namely, it had failed to

- define how, or if, Union Hospital would be represented on the new board.
- define in detail the plan it intended to pursue or how it would be financed.
- circulate a long-range plan as requested.

In summing up, Dreyer wrote: "We consider the new corporation's offer incomplete, its deadline virtually impossible, and its recent statements concerning Union Hospital [as being opposed to the center's goals] incorrect." He emphasized Union's commitment to the concept of a single medical staff by reminding the center that Union had recently invited Truesdale physicians to join the Union staff "with all the same privileges and status they currently have at the Truesdale Hospital." On June 12, 1973, as if to reinforce the message, Union Hospital sent a letter to Truesdale reiterating earlier proposals that the two hospitals consolidate on the Union site.

Meanwhile, Truesdale and Hussey hospitals continued to thrash out the details that would make Fall River Medical and Human Services Center, Inc., a physical reality. In the fall, they filed a determination of need with the state of Massachusetts and Region VII Comprehensive Health Planning, Inc., (HSA). The HSA then sent it to the Fall River Subarea Council of Region Seven, a grassroots citizens' organization, including a minority of hospital representatives, that was charged with evaluating such requests. It

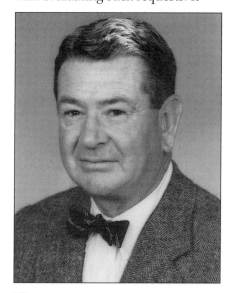

Robert P. Truesdale, chairman, Truesdale Hospital, 1972-1975

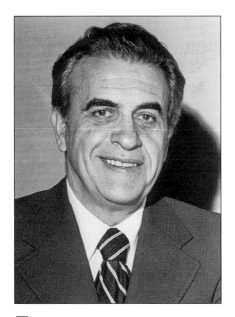

Joseph A. Faria, chairman, Union-Truesdale Hospital, 1975-1976

was here that the buck stopped, and, in effect, "the people" decided the future of Fall River health care.

After an in-depth study, the council concluded Fall River should have one hospital on the north side of the city and one on the south. Saint Anne's was the obvious choice for the south side, with its heavy Catholic population. In the

north, the choice was not yet obvious. But the council did make one thing clear; Truesdale and Union would have to sit down and "plan in earnest." If Union did not bargain in good faith, the council said it would recommend approval of the Truesdale-Hussey merger.

Over most of 1974 Union and Truesdale hospitals engaged in in-depth and often intense negotiating sessions. The pressure to blend two disparate organizations levied an emotional tax on everyone concerned. There also was the matter of strong egos and jockeying for position in the proposed new organization. Dreyer remembers thinking that if conventional wisdom prevailed, he probably would be replaced as administrator. He and his wife, Karen, accepted it as a real possibility. Murray sometimes felt he was unfairly blamed when negotiations stalled. "I resent this becoming known as 'the Murray problem,'" he grumbled at one session. Riding shotgun with

Dreyer and Murray in most sessions were Union trustee George R. Boyce and Truesdale trustee Joseph A. Faria.

During that year, Hussey Hospital gave up the ghost and closed its doors—actually, for not meeting city fire codes. Hussey's programs were shifted from the city hospital to the private sector. This meant that all of its clinics and free-care patients were now the

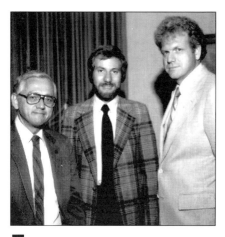

Frederic C. Dreyer, Jr., Union-Truesdale Hospital, president; Arthur J. Sampson, vice-president; Edward M. Klaman, executive vice-president

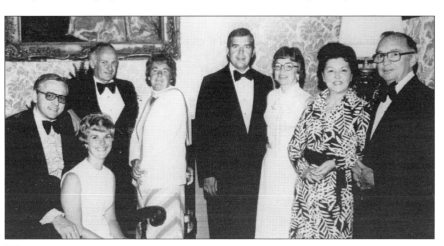

On June 12, 1976, representatives of Union-Truesdale Hospital and St. Anne's Hospital gathered for a formal ball benefiting both institutions. Representing Union-Truesdale were Frederic C. Dreyer, Jr., president and CEO, with Mrs. Dreyer; Robert Murray, director of planning, with Mrs. Murray; and George R. Boyce, chairman of the board, with Mrs. Boyce. Representing St. Anne's were Mrs. Paul A. Giroux and Mr. Giroux, a member of St. Anne's board of trustees.

## Union-Truesdale Hospital in Fall River, Inc.

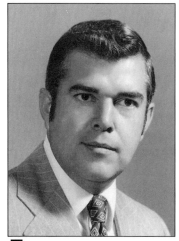

*George R. Boyce, Esq., president, Union-Truesdale Hospital, 1974-1976; chairman, Union-Truesdale Hospital, 1976-1980; chairman, Charlton Memorial Hospital, 1986*

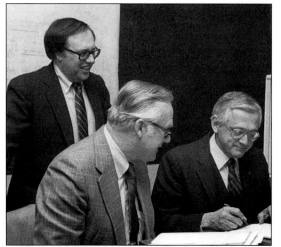

*Carl O. Weaver, systems analyst (later VP); Francis T. Meagher, Esq., Union-Truesdale trustee; and Frederic C. Dreyer, Jr., president, planning for new construction, late 1970s.*

responsibility of the other hospitals. Most of Hussey's former patients were now being cared for at Union's Steven's Clinic. That shortened the equation at the negotiating table but did nothing to ease the pressure. Nevertheless, things were far enough along by October 15 that the Union and Truesdale hospital corporations voted to consolidate. Significantly, Union board president Charles Moran resigned on October 29, to be replaced by Boyce, his younger colleague. By the end of December, Union and Truesdale were ready to file articles of incorporation and a determination of need with the state. It was estimated the review process would take up to eight months.

Finally, on October 1, 1975, the state of Massachusetts issued a charter officially creating the Union-Truesdale Hospital in Fall River, Inc. The long march was over and the future secured. The acute-care facility occupied two sites, boasted 506 beds, and employed 1,700 full- and part-time workers. Perhaps the premiere achievement of the consolidation was the almost seamless transition to a new corporate structure. Almost before the ink had dried, Union-Truesdale was in motion. Plans were launched to

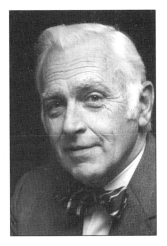

Daniel L. Mooney, MD, trustee and president of Union Hospital medical staff. Dr. Mooney played an important role in the 1975 merger and subsequent development of Charlton Hospital.

# Postconsolidation

In 1975 there were other transitions occurring outside of the consolidation of Union and Truesdale hospitals. The American presence in Vietnam was reduced to a single chaotic rooftop in Saigon, as helicopters ferried civilians away from the invading North Vietnamese. The Organization of Petroleum Exporting Countries, flush with power, raised the price of crude oil by another 10 percent. Nationwide, doctors protested medical malpractice insurance rates, which had quadrupled.

Closer to home, Boston officially launched the American Bicentennial with ceremonies at the Old North Church but did not fare as well in the World Series, losing four games to three to Cincinnati. *Jaws*, a movie about a great white shark terrorizing a New England resort town, proved to be the summer's biggest blockbuster, causing swimmers everywhere to scan the water for menacing fins.

At Union-Truesdale the transition was proceeding smoothly, although not without some "people" hitches. It was one thing to mold a successful corporate structure but quite another to mold hearts and minds. Seventy years of rivalry could not

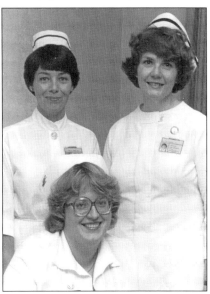

Nurses Arden Dijacomo (sitting), Marcia Liggin and Joan Tralese

consolidate services and departments. The new hospital had not only landed on its feet but at a run.

Frederic C. Dreyer, Jr., was appointed chief executive officer of the new corporation. Other officers for Union-Truesdale were: George R. Boyce, president of the hospital corporation; Joseph A. Faria, chairman of the board of trustees; Robert S. Murray, director of planning and development; William A. Neilan, assistant administrator and treasurer; Everett V. Bradbury, assistant administrator, fiscal analysis; Eleanor E. Presbrey, R.N., assistant administrator, professional services; and F. Bliss Winn, assistant administrator, professional support services. On the medical side, Daniel L. Mooney, M.D., was appointed chief of surgery; William H. Graff, M.D., chief of medicine; and Thomas J. Muldowney, M.D., president of the medical staff.

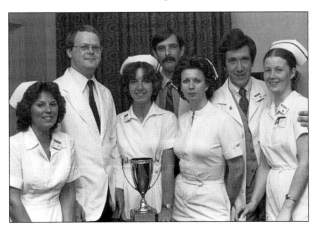

Laurie Palmer, Bob Wilcox, Sue Baulanger, F.S. Gilbert, Mary Wilding, Tom Cinquini, Deb Desmarais, 1979

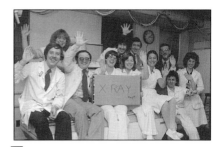

■ *X-ray department 1980*

be erased with the stroke of a pen. Robert S. Murray, who segued from president of Truesdale Hospital to director of planning and development for Union-Truesdale, recalls that several Truesdale people "felt less than welcome" at their new home. In a sense, they also saw fins circling. The strain was nowhere more apparent than among physicians.

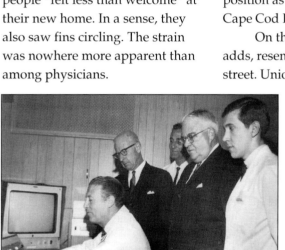

■ *Union Hospital remote control fluroscopy unit upgraded in 1968. Pictured from left to right: Eugene A. Field, MD, chief of radiology; Thomas Hudner, trustee; Robert Semin, MD, associate chief; Lawton S. Brayton, trustee; Thomas Cinquini, department manager.*

Arthur O. Anctil, M.D., a former Union physician who served as medical staff president from 1978 to 1981, reinforces Murray's observations, saying many Truesdale physicians viewed the consolidation as little more than a "hostile takeover." The influence they had exerted at Truesdale disappeared in the Union-Truesdale merger, resulting in considerable friction. Some even moved away. Murray himself remained for five years before accepting a state job and, later, a position as chief operating officer of Cape Cod Hospital.

On the other hand, Anctil adds, resentment was a two-way street. Union doctors simmered over Truesdale debt— much of it unsuspected before consolidation— that was passed on to the new hospital. "As a result of postmerger economic burdens," Anctil says, "capital budgets were restricted for two or three years.

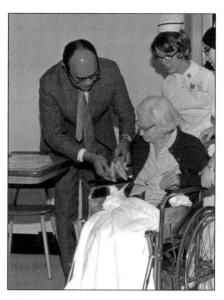

■ *Carl Granger, MD; Bobbie Garvey, RN; and Lana Moniz, RN, work with a patient in the stroke unit at Union, circa early 1970s.*

Union doctors said, 'Hey, it's their fault.'" Anctil recalls bimonthly full staff meetings in which up to a hundred physicians competed to be heard. "It was hard to get anything done," he concedes. By 1980 "things had mellowed out. People began to see that others were not ogres, and there came to be a sense of

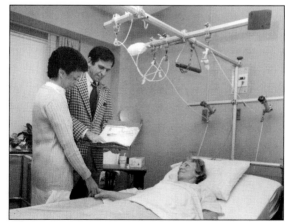

■ *Marge "Fitta" Bockman and Harvey Reback, MD, president of Union Hospital's medical staff, reassure a patient in Brayton 3, circa mid-1970s.*

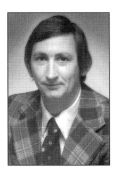

*Thomas J. Muldowney, MD, medical staff president, 1975-1977*

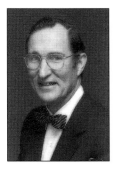

*Philip W. Smith, MD, medical staff president, 1977-1978*

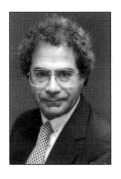

*Arthur O. Anctil, MD, medical staff president, 1978-1981*

camaraderie." A year later, the clamorous full-staff meetings were replaced with streamlined meetings in which physicians sent representatives.

In 1979 Rick Dreyer could report that consolidation of almost all areas of hospital operations have now been completed as planned and hoped for in 1974. Virtually all patient services and operations have been reorganized into single department operations. Everything has been done that can be done until we physically [merge] everything at one location. That year, the Massachusetts Public Health Council approved plans for the site merger. On a more prosaic level employees received a 6 percent pay raise across the board and 120 accruable sick days, doubling the previous number.

In 1982, as site merger loomed, Dreyer pushed hard for more and better outpatient services to meet the challenge of the future. "We must prepare to meet competition between the hospital and outside providers, including 'free-standing,' urgent-care-, and surgery-centers whose activities will increase as the number of physicians increases and the pressures of economic forces cause this ... to intensify." Dreyer proposed experimenting with prepayment concepts, "including possibly" a

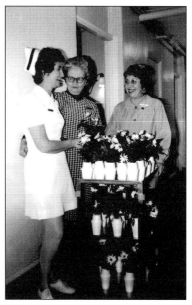

*Jean Quigley, RN, head nurse; May Brimley, director of volunteer services; and Evelyn Lowenstein "Flower Lady," a volunteer who grew flowers at home and routinely distributed flowers to patients for many years*

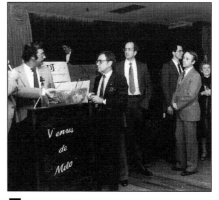

*Physicians present employee awards at the annual employee party. Robert Williamson; Larry Audino, MD; Americo Almeida, MD; Kevin Mabey, MD; Michael King, MD; Rick Schnure, MD; Donna Jean Walker, MD; Robert Delafuente, MD; Frederic C. Dreyer, Jr.*

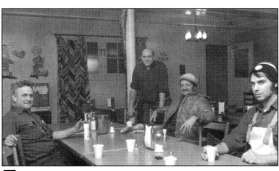

*During the blizzard of 1978 maintenance employees take a break in the Truesdale cafeteria: Louis Pavao, Ken Boyer, Ozzi Guay Paul Tavares.*

hospital-based health maintenance organization.

If there was consolidation tension in the 1970s it did not filter down to the patients. Both Union and Truesdale had built loyal constituencies in the greater Fall River area through the years. Physician names such as Atwood, Mason, Higgins, and Lincoln had become part of the Fall River fabric. If anything, consolidation enhanced that legacy. A 1976 survey of 2,800 discharged patients disclosed that nearly 100 percent rated departments and personnel good to excellent. Even the hospital food—traditionally the butt of bad jokes—received an overwhelmingly favorable rating.

As always those who lost loved ones sent letters of appreciation to the hospital. "On the night that Dad's death was apparent," wrote Robert W. Jean, "your nurses offered us pillows, blankets, coffee, iced tea, and anything else we needed. [They] were so comforting that although we had experienced a great loss, it was somehow made a little easier for us. I am sure your hospital

receives letters of complaints occasionally, so as I promised my Dad, a letter of appreciation was definitely in order. My family will never forget the treatment we received during a very difficult period."

An underplayed though vital component of Union-Truesdale was the hospital chaplaincy program, now called Pastoral Care. It was founded at Union Hospital in 1973 by Rev. Dr. Robert P. Lawrence in cooperation with the Greater Fall River Council of Churches and local hospitals. The chaplaincy program addressed the spiritual needs of patients by providing a ministry away from home. Clergy of all faiths were represented. Lawrence, who later became minister at Fall River's First Congregational Church, also sought to strengthen the healing process through counseling. To those with terminal illnesses he offered understanding and help in

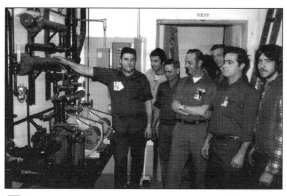

■ *Joe Amaral, Paul Tavares, Louis Pavao, Bob Robinson, Jack Alston, Burt Stockwell, and Allen Ross at the Truesdale site, 1977.*

attaining acceptance.

In 1980 the Reverend David Buehler took over the reins of Pastoral Care, carrying on the ecumenical tradition started by Rev. Lawrence. "Holistic health care begins with the patient and the physician," Buehler said in a 1982 *Pride* interview. "The rest of the team is there to support them." Twenty years earlier, the phrase "holistic health care" might have been considered fringe medicine. Since then, medical science had begun to perceive the healing power of the human mind. Famed

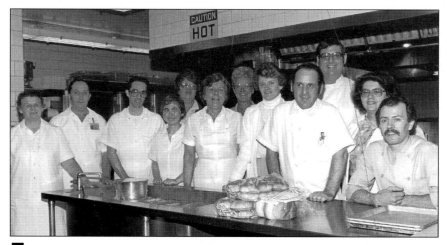

■ *Union-Truesdale kitchen staff: Josephine Rydz, Albino Brasil, Joe Costa, Patty Whelly, Ruth Cadega, Jean Liebl, Del Kiley, Margaret Parmalee, Ronnie Rocha, Jerry Lavoie, Madalin Pimental, John Oliviera*

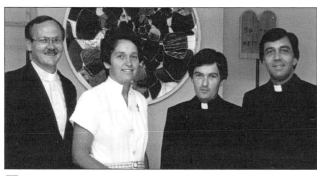

■ *Rev. David Buehler; Sr. Perpetua Lester, RSM; Father George Bellenoit, and Father John Gomes, of Charlton Memorial's Pastoral Care, 1983*

editor Norman Cousins popularized the concept in his best-selling book, *Anatomy of an Illness* (1976), which detailed his own recovery from a serious illness using positive thinking. It was a tribute to the foresight of Union-Truesdale Hospital and its successor, Charlton Memorial Hospital, that not only was the spiritual comfort of patients being nurtured but the untapped healing powers of their minds were, too.

There were other "signs of the times" around the hospital in those postconsolidation years. A nonsmoking policy was established in 1976, a new "restaurant menu" was introduced in 1980, and beepers partially replaced the intercom paging system in 1981. The nonsmoking-policy subcommittee of eleven physicians and employees sought a 1970s-style "fair and equitable" policy that would placate smokers, nonsmokers, and health agencies as well. The "restaurant menu" featured more than thirty entrees, including restricted diets. Food was now cooked in small quantities to enhance freshness and prevent waste—a kitchen precursor to total quality management. Thanks to beepers, the hospital became quieter and more responsive. Unlike the intercom, beepers could be heard in elevators, tunnels, and air-conditioned offices.

Between 1974 and 1980, several members of the "old guard" departed the scene. Manual "Manny" Carvalho, chief engineer at Union for forty years, retired in 1974, while Madison F. Welsh, clerk of the Union Hospital Corporation, stepped down a year later after fifty years on the board. In 1976 Alma Janson, R.N., retired after forty-six years at Union as OR supervisor and central-supply manager. She was followed in 1977 by Eleanor E.

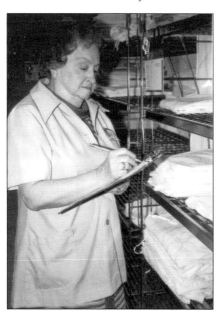

■ *Angelia Jeanrichard was supervisor of the hospital's laundry for fifty-six years.*

Presbrey, director of nursing for thirty-three years, and Angie Jeanrichard, supervisor of laundry and linen distribution, who wrapped up fifty-six years at Union. John B. Cummings, former Truesdale trustee and president of the board, died in 1978. His death was followed two years later by George M. Jackson, former Union administrator.

# Growing Pains

*I*n 1979 Union-Truesdale Hospital finally embarked on a long anticipated construction project after a frustrating delay of twenty-two months in obtaining a determination of need. Board chairman John Dator finally convinced the Massachusetts Public Health Council that any more delay would only inflate costs and burden taxpayers. The new Y-

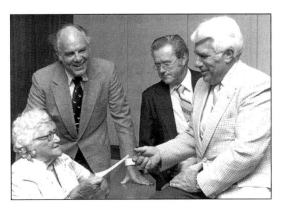

Mrs. Warren Atwood presents a donation to Charlton Memorial Hospital (from left) William Murray, William Neilan, and Rev. Dr. Robert Lawrence.

shaped, five-story building, designed by Karlsberg & Associates of Columbus, Ohio, would encompass 156,724 square feet and be called the Atwood Building, after the late, beloved Truesdale physician Warren G. Atwood. It would house new emergency, radiology, and outpatient departments, and intensive- and progressive-care units plus 192 single-patient-care units.

With its optimal use of hospital space, the Atwood Building represented a new concept

in health care. Most hospitals did not have single-patient care units, which reduced the need to transfer patients and allowed them to be placed without regard to sex, diagnosis, or age. The result was shortened hospital stays. The completion of the Atwood Building would weld the hospital to one site and spell the demise of Truesdale as a hospital.

Before the first spade could be turned, there was the matter of funding to consider. In the end, the project would cost $37 million. Most of that would be paid through long-term financing. To qualify for such financing, Union-Truesdale hospital would be obligated to raise a substantial sum on its own. That figure, which was set at $5 million, would be obtained from fund drives targeting the hospital and the community. The hospital would lead the way. If employees, staff, and auxiliary responded generously, it was reasoned, so would the community.

The initial chairman of the Union-Truesdale building-fund campaign was Kenneth List, who died in the early stages of the drive. He was replaced by John F. Dator, chairman of the board of trustees. Other fund-drive leaders included Ken Boyer, assistant chief engineer and employees division chairman; Sheila Salvo, auxiliary president; and Dr.

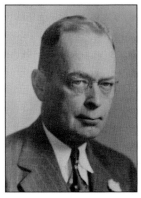

Warren G. Atwood, MD, president, Truesdale Hospital, 1943-1946

Anctil. The fund drive began in June 1979 and concluded in October 1980. In between, a task force of some two hundred employees and numerous volunteers contributed thousands of hours to the cause. Employees were asked to pledge thirty minutes of their pay per week over a three-year period, but Boyer emphasized that participation was prized more than money. "Participation," he said, "will have a solid impact on what the community will do."

As the fund drive kicked off, Rick Dreyer and the Rev. Dr.

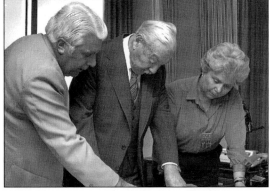

Rev. Dr. Robert P. Lawrence, director of development(left) and Jane Babiarz, director of marketing (right) for Charlton Memorial Hospital present plans for the Atwood Building to philanthropist William List in his New York offices, early 1980s.

Robert Lawrence were quietly concluding a mission to rekindle a relationship that had been dormant for a generation. The Charlton family, who had contributed so much moral and financial support to the Truesdale and Union hospitals in earlier years, had gradually shifted its philanthropic focus to the Mayo Clinic in Rochester, Minnesota. In fact, Ruth Charlton Mitchell Masson, daughter of Woolworth cofounder Earle P. Charlton, lived there full-time.

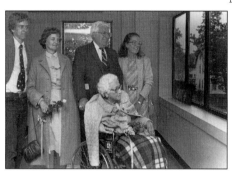

■ *Drs. Elizabeth Atwood Lawrence and Rev. Robert Lawrence with their son, Mark, and daughter, Priscilla, tour Leila Atwood through the new Atwood Building dedicated to the memory of her husband, Warren G. Atwood, MD.*

■ *Charlton Memorial Hospital Board of Trustees–1980*
*Front Row: Robert E. Hutton, treasurer; Paul V. Stevens, vice president; Atty. George R. Boyce, president; John F. Dator, chairman; Donald H. Ramsbottom, vice president; George M. Jackson, former clerk and administrator; Clement J. Dowling, clerk.*
*Second Row: Russell R. Harmon; Ruth Merritt; Sanford W. Udis, MD; Neilson M. Caplain; Janet Edmonds; Ruth E. Hurley; Sheila Salvo, president of the auxiliary; William M. Hoban; Robert S. Murray, director of planning and development.*
*Third Row: Philemon E. Truesdale; F. Robert Laing; Donald L. Walker; Arthur K. Smith, MD, trustee; William H. Graff, MD, trustee; Carl R. Larkin; Thomas F. Cooney; Atty. Francis T. Meagher; Daniel L. Mooney, MD; Arthur O. Anctil, MD, president of the medical staff; Frederic C. Dreyer, Jr., administrator and CEO*

Dreyer gives credit to Rev. Dr. Lawrence for playing the central role in the rapprochement, which resulted in a $1 million contribution to the building fund and the renaming of Union-Truesdale to Charlton Memorial Hospital. Dreyer and Rev. Dr. Lawrence made several trips to Rochester to reestablish links with Mrs. Masson, then in her late eighties, and update her on hospital progress. On behalf of the hospital board, trustee Donald Ramsbottom also established rapport with Mrs. Masson and paid a visit. With utmost skill and diplomacy, he delineated the volunteer dimension of the hospital and system.

"Bob Lawrence's wife, Betty, was like a daughter to Mrs. Masson," Dreyer said. "As the daughter of Dr. Warren G. Atwood, a highly respected Fall River physician and Charlton family favorite, she visited Mrs. Masson every summer at her horse farm in Pennsylvania." Dr. Elizabeth Atwood Lawrence recalls that Mrs. Masson "didn't

have any children, so she sort of adopted me. We had a very close friendship throughout the years." The same was true of Rev. Dr. Lawrence, whom Mrs. Masson viewed as her personal minister. "He flew up there several times a year to be with her," Dreyer said.

Dreyer remembers Mrs. Masson as "very demanding,

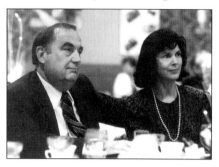

■ *Earle P. Charlton, II and his wife, Frances, at the dedication of the Atwood Building, 1983*

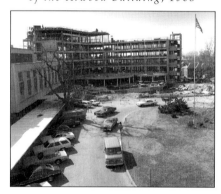

■ *Construction of the Atwood Building, 1982*

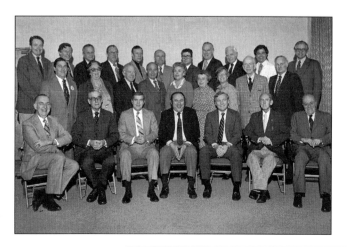

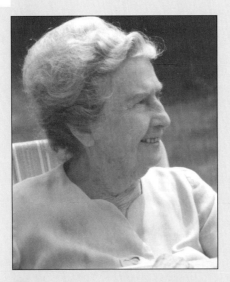

*Ruth Charlton Mitchell Masson during her visit to Charlton Memorial in the early 1980s after she contributed the first $1 million to the capital campaign to build the Atwood Building.*

## Ruth Charlton Mitchell Masson

During a life span that reached 104 years, Ruth Charlton Mitchell Masson bore witness to incredible changes. When she was born, a German named Otto Lilienthal made news by strapping on crude wings and gliding a few feet off the ground. When she died, astronauts were manning space stations for months at a time while unmanned satellites hurtled past Jupiter.

The oldest of three children born to Earle P. Charlton, a cofounder of the Woolworth retail empire, Ruth was the sibling most actively involved in the family philanthropies. It was Ruth who oversaw the creation of facilities, research grants, and scholarships at the Mayo Clinic. It was Ruth who consented to reestablish ties with Fall River in the late 1970s after a hiatus of twenty years and contributed $1 million to the building fund of Union-Truesdale— now Charlton—Hospital. And it is Ruth's name that graces the Ruth Charlton Mitchell Therapies Center, a multi dimensional Fall River facility that opened in 1992.

She was born in 1891 in Fall River during the heyday of the textile industry. For the daughter of a rising business tycoon, life was good in Spindle City. In 1911 she was one of eighteen young women chosen for the queen's court in the Cotton Centennial. Three years later, she married Frederick Mitchell, a leather merchant from Philadelphia, in a lavish wedding Fall River newspapers described as a "fairy-tale."

Ruth and "Fritz" (as friends called him) built a luxurious home in Westport. Years later the house was destroyed by the New England hurri-

cane of 1938. In between, they purchased Fox Valley farm in Pennsylvania and Mandalay fishing lodge in Maine. The couple, who had no children, lived life to the fullest as they traveled, raised horses, and made fishing excursions. Mrs. Masson also was a tennis buff. Retired Fall River architect Anthony Waring, whose parents, Ruth and Ellis, were good friends of the Mitchells, recalls "Aunt Ruth" as a "very correct and proper" woman who once sent him a crate of pigeons when she discovered he had an interest in raising them.

Waring remembers "Uncle Fritz" as a jovial "Wallace Beery type" who often went fishing with his father and Dr. Warren Atwood of Truesdale Hospital. When his friends caught bigger fish, Mitchell was wont to hurl his rod and reel into the lake, then get new equipment back at camp. "He always stocked up at L.L. Bean on the way up," Waring explained. Once, when his car broke down on a road trip, Mitchell, a solutions-oriented sort, bought a new one on the spot and continued his journey.

Over the years, Ruth developed a deep and abiding friendship with Dr. Atwood's daughter, Elizabeth—now Elizabeth Atwood Lawrence, V.M.D.— who began visiting the Pennsylvania farm at age five. Lawrence recalls that Ruth organized treasure hunts and arranged horseback rides chaperoned by the farm foreman. She remembers being amazed at "how clean the pigs were." Lawrence credits those childhood years at Ruth Mitchell's farm with playing a major role in her later decision to become a veterinarian.

By all accounts, the Mitchells were devoted to each other. "He liked to needle her in a friendly way," Waring says of Fritz Mitchell. But this was obviously more than a marriage of social convenience. The Mitchells understood each other and—in certain ways—were alike. For example, Ruth once was persuaded to fly to Fall River, even though she had never flown before and feared aircraft. As luck would have it, the plane developed engine trouble and had to land. In a "Fritz redux" scenario, she went to a car dealer and bought a Cadillac on the spot. She never flew again.

In 1960 "Fritz" died, ending a marriage of forty-six years. Five years later, Ruth married Dr. William Masson, a Mayo Clinic physician and old family friend. Fall River's Rev. Dr. Robert Lawrence conducted the service. For the remaining thirty years of her life, she resided in Rochester, Minnesota.

On February 11, 1995, Ruth Charlton Mitchell Masson died at the age of 104 years. A memorial service officiated by Rev. Dr. Robert P. Lawrence at the First Congregational Church in Fall River overflowed with physicians, nurses, and local residents. Employees from the hospital made a human chain around the hospital to watch the funeral procession as it left for the Oak Grove Cemetery. By order of the mayor, all flags in Fall River were flown at half-mast.

But the Charlton legacy lives on, due in no small measure to this remarkable woman who kept aloft the torch of generosity handed down by her father. ▆

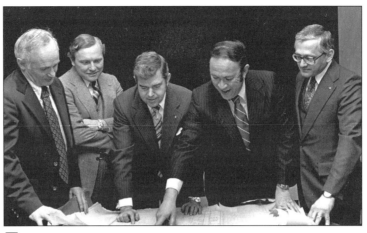

Robert S. Murray, former president of Truesdale Hospital; Donald H. Ramsbottom, chairman of Union-Truesdale; George R. Boyce, former chairman of Union; John F. Dator, trustee of Union-Truesdale; and Frederic C. Dreyer, Jr., president of Union-Truesdale plan the Atwood Building, circa early 1980s.

professional, polite, and cordial." Others recall her as a strong-willed woman who "knew her place," which was on the top rung of the ladder. Yet her instinct for doing the right thing was unerring. "We encouraged her to visit Fall River," recalls Dreyer, who with Rev. Dr. Lawrence, trustees, physicians, and old friends showed her around Union-Truesdale Hospital. "She hadn't been here for fourteen years." As she was leaving, she called Dreyer and Lawrence over to her car. "Call Mr. Dodge [her personal banker] at the First National Bank of Boston," she said. "He'll be expecting your call." Up went the power window, and she was gone.

The Union-Truesdale Board of Trustees, under the leadership of trustee John F. Dator, set a $5 million capital fund-raising goal. The board fired the fund-raising consultant, who said the goal was unachievable in Fall River, and the

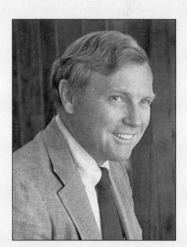

Donald H. Ramsbottom, chairman, Charlton Memorial Hospital, 1980-1985 chairman, Charlton Health System, 1983-1986

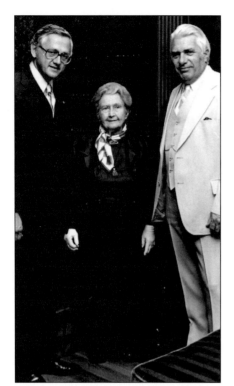

Frederic C. Dreyer, Jr.; Ruth Charlton Mitchell Masson; and Rev. Dr. Robert Lawrence

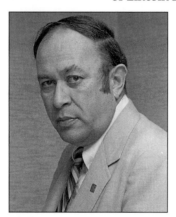

John F. Dator, president, Union-Truesdale Hospital, 1976-1978 chairman, Union-Truesdale Hospital/Charlton Memorial Hospital, 1978-1980 chairman, Charlton Memorial Hospital Foundation, Inc., 1988-1992

campaign proceeded. The Charlton family pledge of $1 million was announced in September 1979. This contribution pushed the fund drive to $2.3 million, almost halfway to the goal. A *Pride* article recalled how, through the terms of his will, E.P. Charlton had provided perpetual endowment funds for Union and Truesdale hospitals. It recalled how his widow, Ida, and children, Ruth, Earle P. Jr. ("Perry"), and Virginia, had continued to support the medical community in Fall River.

It recalled, for example, Ruth's contribution of the Ida S. Charlton Library at Truesdale Hospital, Perry Charlton's generosity in keeping Truesdale equipped with ambulances, and Virginia Lincoln's gift to Truesdale of Lincoln Pediatrics. It was Virginia, in fact, who presented every newborn baby at Truesdale with a layette. The article reminded readers that Ruth's first husband, Frederick M. Mitchell, had faithfully served as trustee and president of the Truesdale board for many years. Clearly, the Charlton family's Fall River roots were long and deep and deserving of lasting recognition.

On March 1, 1980, Union-Truesdale Hospital was renamed Charlton Memorial Hospital. At dedication ceremonies, Earle P. Charlton, II, grandson of the family patriarch, described his grandfather as an adventurer and innovator. The younger Charlton, a successful Woolworth executive and entrepreneur himself, recently had been tapped to assist his aunt in overseeing the Charlton family philanthropies. "I went to work for Woolworth right out of college," he recalls, "and worked my way up to regional manager and vice president of the Pacific region. I think my aunt felt I had put in my time." The hospital's name change not only honored the Charlton family, it struck a neutral tone that softened old rivalries.

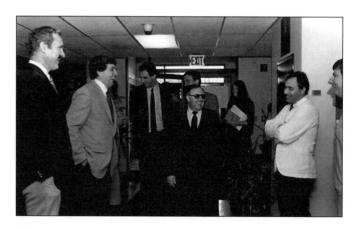

Robert McDonald, Senator Thomas Norton, Kenneth Fiola, Carl Weaver (with glasses), John Gurney, and Robert Turgeon tour Charlton Memorial.

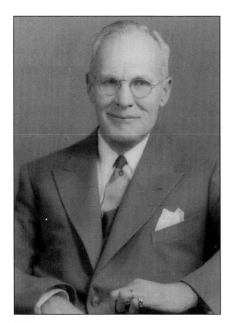

*Frederick M. Mitchell, president, Truesdale Hospital, 1922-1924*

By August the fund drive stood at $4.5 million, thanks to a $250,000 contribution from the Donaldson Foundation of New York. By November 26, the drive was over, and groundbreaking ceremonies commenced. Charlton employees had contributed $300,000, while the auxiliary and the Charlton medical staff chipped in $500,000 each. The remainder came from community and corporate pledges. It was the largest single fund drive in Fall River history.

The ensuing construction and site merger proved to be a logistical challenge of the first order. In addition to the excavation, the trucks, and the stockpiles of material, some two hundred workers milled about the premises. In fact, construction so interfered with traffic that the emergency room had to be relocated into the Borden Building during

# E.P. "Chuck" Charlton, II

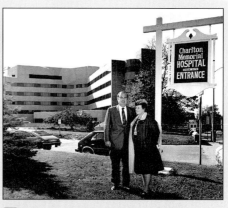

*Earle P. Charlton, II, and his sister, Thelma C. West, 1983*

E.P. "Chuck" Charlton, II, the son of E.P. Charlton, Jr., and grandson of E.P. Charlton, was born in West Newton, a suburb of Boston, and raised in Nevada. During the summers, Chuck and his sister, Thelma, vacationed at "Pond Meadow," the palatial Charlton estate at Westport Harbor. At the age of seventeen, Chuck Charlton enlisted in the U.S. Navy and spent several months during World War II as a naval-recognition expert spotting German submarines in the Caribbean. After the war, he earned a college degree at the University of Nevada and went to work for the Woolworth chain at an entry-level position.

Charlton spent twenty-nine years with Woolworth, ending his career as regional manager and vice president of the Pacific region, which included thirteen western states, Hawaii, and Alaska. Later, he participated in the starting of the popular Ross Clothing chain and Bookmania, a chain of discount bookstores.

It wasn't until the mid-1980s that Ruth Charlton Mitchell Masson invited him to participate in the management of the Charlton family trusts. Until then, his links with the family had been sporadic. "I think Ruth admired the fact that I went to work for Woolworth right out of college," he says. "I think she felt I had put in my time."

Charlton recalls that when his father died, he left nearly all of his estate—some $8 million—to charity. During his lifetime, he made it a point to keep Truesdale Hospital supplied with the latest ambulances.

Although Charlton made his home in Hillsborough, California, where he lives with his wife Frances and their daughter Stacey, he continues to keep close ties with Charlton Memorial Hospital and Charlton Health System as a trustee and later as trustee emeritus of Southcoast Hospital Group.

He also remains active as trustee of the Charlton Charitable Trusts which primarily benefit medical programs, research, hospitals and education throughout the state of Massachusetts with special emphasis on southeastern Massachusetts. His personal philanthropic efforts also extend throughout California and Nevada.

In 1996 the University of Massachusetts Dartmouth presented Charlton with the honorary degree of Doctor of Business Administration.

Early in 1997 Charlton announced that the new College of Business and Industry at UMass Dartmouth would be named for his grandfather, Earle Perry Charlton. ■

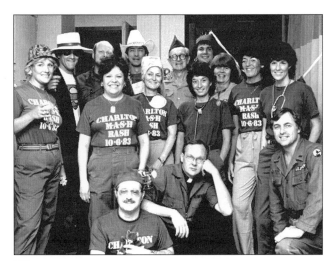

On October 6, 1983, during cafeteria renovations, Charlton held a "MASH BASH" look alike contest. First Place Winners (back row): Elaine Phillibert as Major Margaret "Hot Lips" Houlihan; John Quatramoni, MD as Capt. B.J. Hunnicut; Paul Collard as Major Charles Emerson Winchester, III; Steve Roy as Capt. Benjamin Franklin "Hawkeye" Pierce; Walter Dugan as Col. Sherman Potter; Bob Cunha as Corp. Maxwell Klinger. Second Place Winners (middle row): Fran Turgeon as Nurse Kelly; Joyce Beauchaine, RN; Maureen Camara, RN; Roberta Stemiza; Sharon Carmichael; Colleen Driscoll. Third Place Winners (Bottom): Dave "Rocky" Ferreira as Corp. Walter "Radar" O'Reilly; Rev. David Buehler as Father Francis Mulcahy; and John Gurney

construction. Another formidable task involved transporting the heavy equipment of the radiology and diagnostic-imaging departments from Truesdale to Union. It took four months, which might not have been the case if Charlton had been a conventional business. But a hospital has to be fully functional regardless of circumstances. Everything had to be planned with military precision. Equipment and personnel had to end up in the right place at the right time. It could have been a matter of life and death.

Another problem during the building period was lack of parking spaces. The original number of 403 slots was devoured by an omnivorous construction site. In April 1981 *Pride* assured Charlton employees that 268 more slots would be added by the end of summer and an additional 108 spaces in the fall. According to Kenneth Kiley, Sr., project representative for the hospital, the parking lots were being carved out of property where houses had been razed or moved. Dreyer estimates some twelve houses were moved to make room for the Atwood Building. The houses were purchased by Charlton, which offered them to buyers for a pittance if they would pay to have them relocated. Seven homes were relocated. When the project was completed, Charlton employees sighed with relief. More than nine hundred parking spaces had been created.

On May 27, 1983, the Warren G. Atwood, M.D., Patient Care Facility, popularly known as Atwood Tower, was dedicated. The last patients from Truesdale were

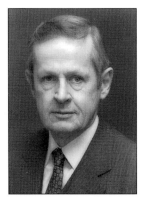

Francis M. James, MD, medical staff president, 1981-1982

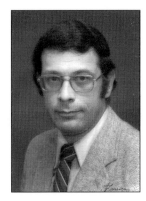

Lawrence F. Audino, MD, medical staff president, 1983-1985

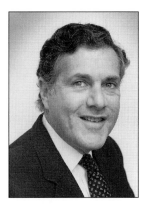

Herbert S. Rubin, MD, medical staff president, 1985-1988

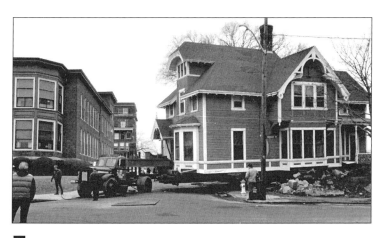

■ *Relocating the house belonging to Stephen Nawrocki to make way for hospital expansion, March 1982.*

scheduled to arrive at Charlton within two weeks, just before ancillary services there were shut down. Its work done, Truesdale Hospital would slip into history. The complex strategic plan to physically consolidate all activities into one site, depicted on a wall-sized PERT (Performance Evaluation Review Technique) Chart in Rick Dreyer's office, was now accomplished and on schedule. Now as champagne corks popped inside the yellow-and-white striped tent and colored balloons hugged the canvas ceiling, Leila Atwood, the white-haired widow of Dr. Atwood, sat quietly in a wheelchair. Outside, the sky was overcast.

Among those present was Charlton's Dr. Sidney W. Rosen, who had been a close friend of Dr. Atwood's. "I met him just after my discharge from the navy following World War II," Dr. Rosen recalls. "Like other young men, I was drawn to him by his charisma. He was 'The Chief,' and we tried to emulate him." During the war, when civilian doctors were scarce, Dr. Atwood was delivering approximately two

thousand babies a year on top of a full surgical schedule. "I think he pushed so hard that it contributed to his contracting tuberculosis," Dr. Rosen said. Atwood also was an avid medical historian, who liked to collect early papers on the uses of ether. He was the "epitome of a physician"—a man who related well to his patients and possessed great clinical skills. Dr. Rosen knows this first hand, "He delivered my own daughter," he added.

Earle P. Charlton II spoke of how proud his grandfather would have been of the hospital that now bore his name. U.S. secretary of health and human services

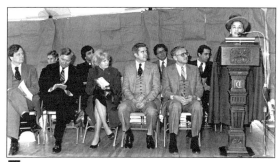

■ *The Atwood Building dedication on May 27, 1983. Rev. Donald Meir; State Rep. Joan Menard; Donald H. Ramsbottom, Charlton Memorial board chairman; Rev. John Gomes; Margaret Heckler, secretary of HEW; George R. Boyce, Esq.; Arthur Anctil, MD; Frederic C. Dreyer, Jr., president of Charlton Memorial Hospital; Carlton Viveiros, mayor; and State Sen. Mary Fonseca (speaking)*

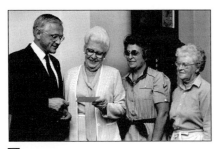

*Members of the Truesdale Nurses Alumnae Association present a donation to the Charlton Memorial Development Fund to Frederic C. Dreyer, Jr. Proceeds were donated from a farewell party held at the closing of the Truesdale site. Dolores "Del" Crispo, RN, chairman of the event; Linda Machado, RN, chairman of reservations committee; and Sybil C. Anderson, RN, chairman of the memorabilia committee, August 1983.*

Margaret Heckler applauded the crowd for taking action in providing "more efficient and high quality services." Donald H. Ramsbottom, chairman of the board of trustees, urged expansion of outpatient services. And Rick Dreyer peered into the future again when he suggested Charlton should link with other hospitals in southeastern Massachusetts to form a regional health care system.

Two years later, the new infill building between Elizabeth House and the Brayton Building was dedicated as the Ruth C. and Frederick M. Mitchell Building. Ceremonies took place in the Ida S. Charlton Library, which had been moved from Truesdale Hospital and faithfully recreated in the new medical-education complex on the first floor. The second floor housed an expanded obstetrics department that included seven labor-delivery-recovery rooms, two standard delivery rooms, three term nurseries, an isolation nursery, a Level II special-care nursery, and a post partum unit comprising twenty-eight private rooms. Ruth (Mitchell) Masson participated in ceremonies

by phone from her home in Rochester. Others in attendance included Dr. Elizabeth Atwood Lawrence; her mother Leila Atwood; and Earle P. Charlton, II.

In July Truesdale Hospital was sold for $370,000 to developer James Karam and the Claremont Company of New Bedford. The hospital where charismatic Philemon Truesdale roamed the halls and Alice McHenry underwent her famous "upside-down" stomach operation would become a home for the elderly. Perhaps some of the new residents would gaze down at the Taunton River from time to time and remember. ■

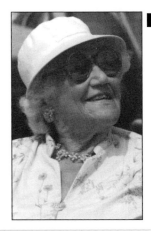

*Mrs. Leila Atwood, circa 1980s*

## CMH Auxiliary Stays the Course

From the turn of the century to the 1990s, the Charlton Memorial Hospital Auxiliary (formerly Women's Board) has never altered its mission, which is to raise money for the institution and serve as ambassadors to the community. In earlier times, the organization provided a socially acceptable way for women to wield influence in the community without stepping out of the cultural role assigned to them. In more recent years, the auxiliary has abandoned its gender camouflage in favor of a more neutral image, as witnessed by the name change and the fact that 5 percent of the membership is now men.

For many years, the CMH Auxiliary produced the annual follies, a rustic affair featuring such hijinks as men—often including physicians—dancing the can-can. Since 1995, the auxiliary has opted for more sedate events such as theme parties. In 1996 the auxiliary hosted six hundred people and netted $24,000 at the Fall Fantasy gala. The previous year's event had garnered $20,000. The 1996 theme party was described as "upscale and elegant with ballroom dancing and food stations."

Another major annual event is the Spring Luncheon, where four health-career scholarships of $1,000 each are presented to recipients from Charlton Memorial Hospital, Bristol Community College, and the University of Massachusetts at Dartmouth. At the yearly Dinner Luncheon a check for $100,000 on average is given to the hospital administration, enlarging a $1 million endowment pledged in 1990.

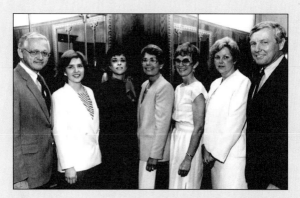

Frederic C. Dreyer, Jr. (left) and Donald H. Ramsbottom (right) with auxiliary board members 1985: Linda Monchik, Carolyn Kaiser, Patricia Bartek, Marcia Zuehlke, Sandra Booth

Separate but equal to the auxiliary is the Charlton Volunteer organization. Where the auxiliary focuses on fundraising, the volunteers donate their labor—they staff the gift shop, and the information desk, push the book carts, and, in general, perform a variety of chores for Charlton. Over the years, volunteers have gone about their business without fanfare. The services they have provided and wages they have saved have contributed in no small measure to Charlton's reputation as a premiere medical institution. "For one hundred years," says Carol O'Connell, former chairman of the Charlton board of trustees, "volunteers have devoted thousands of hours to the hospital. They are to be commended."

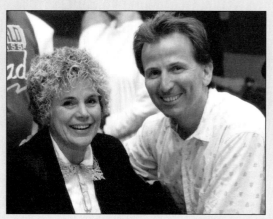

Carol A. O'Connell, chair of the 1991 follies chats with Raymond Audet who decorated props for the fund-raiser.

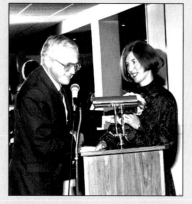

Frederic C. Dreyer, Jr. presents an appreciation award to Carole Waxler, president of the auxiliary.

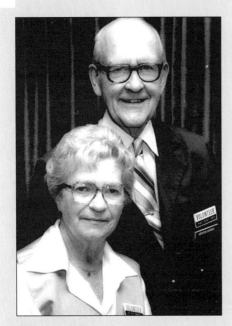

*Long-time volunteers Mr. and Mrs. Newton Skinner*

Rick Dreyer, former president and chief executive officer of Charlton Memorial Hospital and Charlton Health System, agrees. "The auxiliary and volunteers, more than anyone, embody the voluntary spirit of Charlton. They comprise people of greater Fall River and of the Charlton system. The success of Charlton depends on their support." The auxiliary currently counts 340 members. Direct service volunteers number 260 members. Dreyer continued, "People like Cid Mahoney and Debra Curless, past and present directors of volunteers, have done a remarkable job of constantly influencing and helping volunteers to identify and implement volunteer avenues of service. Generations of volunteer leaders and workers, more than anything else, have kept the volunteer spirit alive and viable at Charlton."

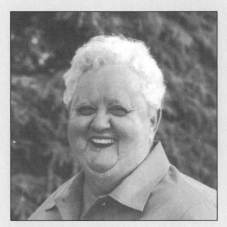

*Marion Lincoln has been a volunteer for over ten years and has given over 3,000 hours. She prefers to give her time at the information desk where she has helped hundreds of people in moments of crisis. When asked about her volunteering experiences she replied, "It is a thrill to be involved in this institution and its mission of serving others."-Photo by Jack Foley at* The Fall River Herald News.

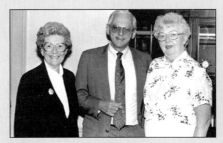

*Cecilia Mahoney, director of volunteer services; Frederic C. Dreyer, Jr.; and Claire Thompson, auxiliary president*

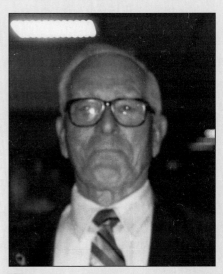

*Mr. Earnest W. Bell was police chief in Swansea, Massachusetts for twenty years. In his eighteen years since retirement, he has volunteered at Charlton over nineteen thousand hours.*

C

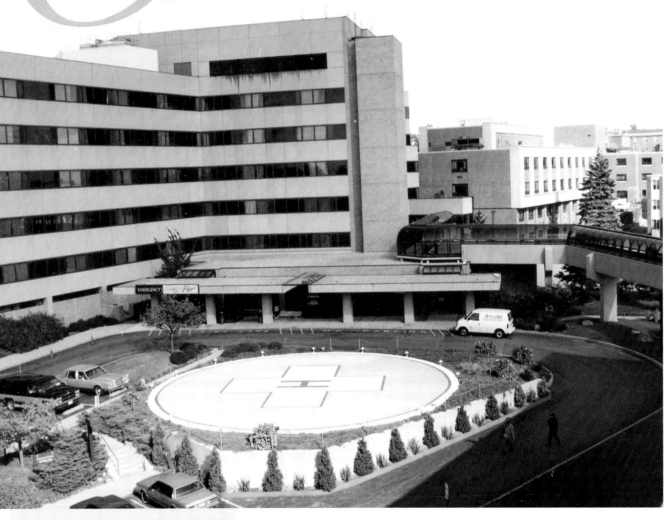

*E R   e n t r a n c e ,   O c t o b e r   1 9 9 2*

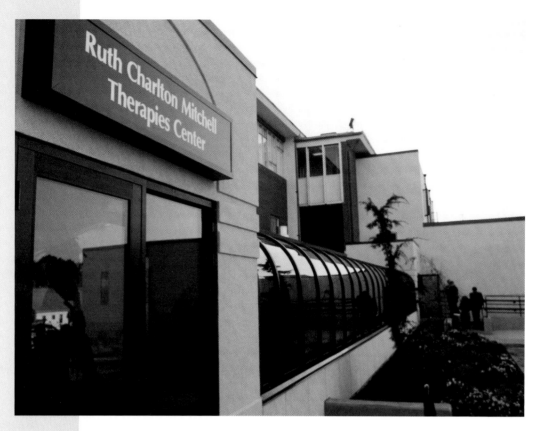

*The Ruth Charlton Mitchell Therapies Center opened in 1992.*

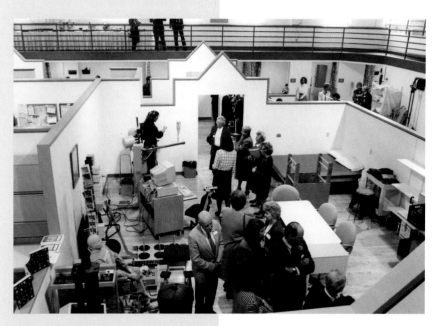

*The Ruth Charlton Mitchell Therapies Center features areas for numerous types of therapies.*

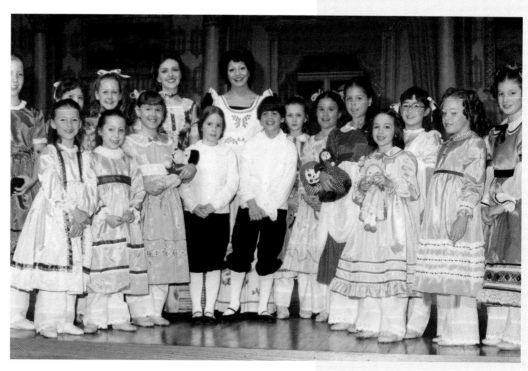

On December 1 and 2, 1979, the Auxiliary presented "The Nutcracker" involving local talent to raise money for the hospital.

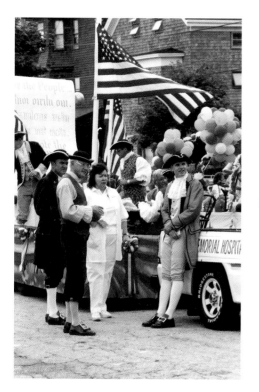

Charlton employees' float in the "Fall River Celebrates America" parade, foreground: George Lesure, vice president of human resources; Frederic C. Dreyer, Jr., president of CHS and CHM; Lynn Davis, RN, clinical director of nursery services; E. Tod Allen, vice president of strategic planning

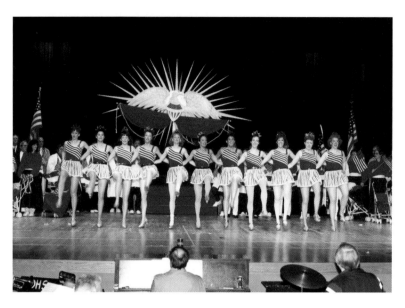

*"What's a follies without a chorus line?" at the 1991 follies*

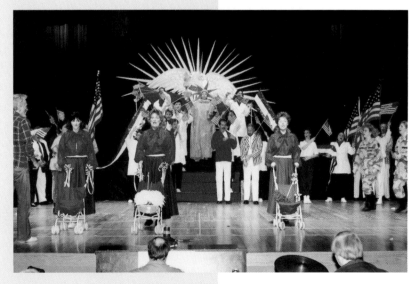

*Follies continued to be popular fund-raisers into the 1980s, foreground: Lois Spirlet, Nancy Dineen, Marcia Liggin.*

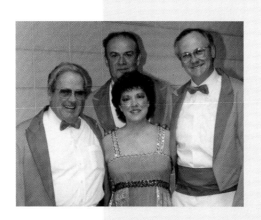

eorge Lesure, director of human
sources; Rev. David Buehler;
obert Bellefuille, security; and
ucille Poirier, cancer registry
se prior to their stage debut at
e 1991 follies.

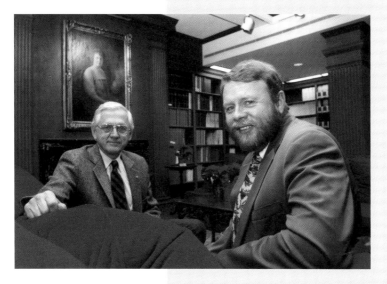

Frederic C. Dreyer, Jr.,
president of Charlton Health
System with Ronald B.
Goodspeed, MD, who became the
new president of Charlton
Memorial Hospital effective
January 1, 1995.

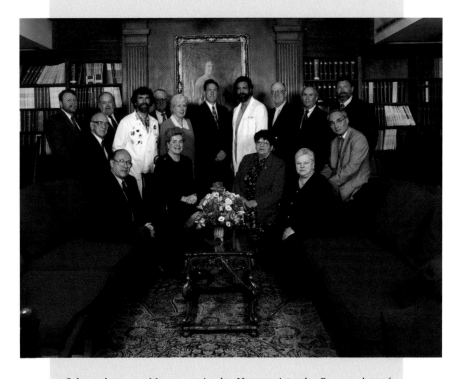

*Charlton Memorial Hospital Board of Trustees 1996, (sitting, front): John F. Dator; Carol A. O'Connell, immediate past chairman; Rita N. Wood, clerk; Elisabeth Pennington; (second row, sitting/standing): Ronald B. Goodspeed, MD, president; Paul S. Vaitses, Jr.; John C. Corrigan, Jr., Esq; Stephen S. Kasparian, MD; Francis M. James, MD; Eileen T. Farley, first vice chairman; William H. Lapointe, chairman; William L. Kasdon, MD; William J. Torpey; Joseph F. Motta, Ed.D.; Jay S. Schachne, MD; Peter D. Kane (seated); (not present): Earle P. Charlton, II; Frederic C. Dreyer, Jr., ex-officio; George S. Smith, Ed.D.; Paula Raposa, second vice chairman*

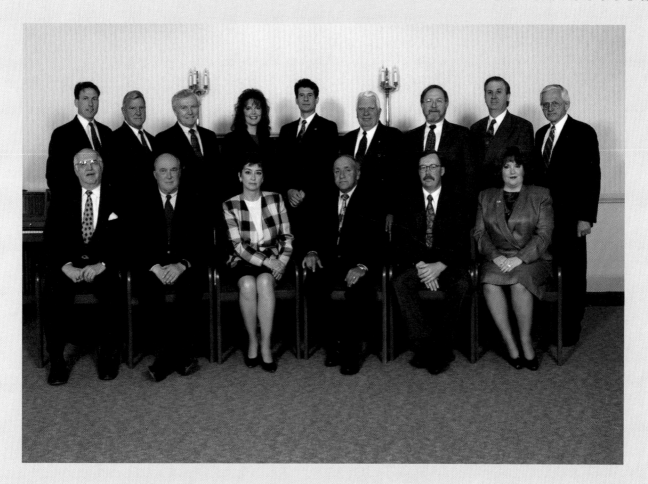

Charlton Health System Board of Trustees 1996, (sitting): Arthur Marchand, Jr., clerk; Barry Robbins, past chairman; Agatha St. Amour; John M. Almeida, chairman; James M. Worthington, MD, second vice chairman; Emily Myles; (standing): William H. Lapointe; Daniel E. Bogan; Donald H. Ramsbottom; Tracy R. Greene; Russell Guerreiro; Rev. Dr. Robert P. Lawrence; Ronald A. Schwartz, MD; Paul Beaulieu; Frederic C. Dreyer, Jr., president; (not present): Earle P. Charlton, II, trustee emeritus

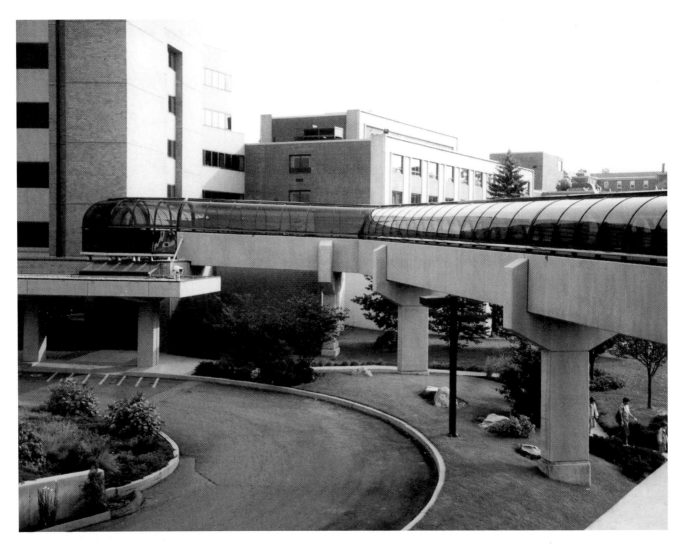

*A new walkway connected the parking garage to the hospital in 1995*

# Into the Future

# *Chapter Five*

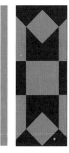

With the completion of the Atwood and Mitchell buildings, Charlton Memorial Hospital was ready for the next leg of its journey. Now that it had a modern and expansive infrastructure, hospital leadership could concentrate on developing new programs and services for its greater Fall River patients. It could focus on more sophisticated technology, which offered procedures undreamed of a scant few years before. It could refine outpatient concepts in ways that would counteract the rising costs of medicine and yet provide superior services. And it could explore new medical opportunities to meet changing times. Donald Ramsbottom, Charlton board of trustees chairman, described the emerging scene in the annual report for 1983:

> If a hospital is to survive, it must become competitive and realize that it is now, to a certain degree, a part of our free enterprise system. From

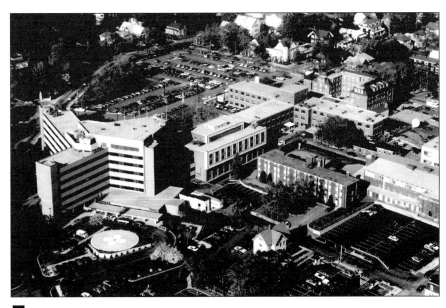

*Aerial, early 1990s*

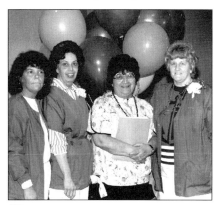

*Madeline Furtado, Cindy Boucher, Rita Wood, and Marie Lopes. Rita Wood, trustee, speaks to secretaries on Secretaries Day 1989*

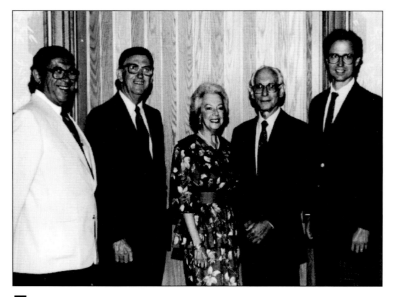

John Dator; William Torpey; Ruth Resnick; Albert Resnick, MD; and Rick Schnure, MD, at Dr. Resnick's retirement party

freestanding clinics to HMOs, to surgicenters and competitive organizations, a hospital today must do its own marketing if it is to grow and survive.

Ramsbottom's succinct appraisal echoed the historical vision and sensitivity to community needs manifested by the board since the turn of the century. It had begun with Union Hospital's John D. Flint and been carried on by Richard P. Borden, John S. Brayton, and Charles M. Moran. Truesdale Hospital ran parallel with leaders such as Philemon Truesdale, M.D.; Ralph W. French, M.D.; E.P. Charlton; Warren G. Atwood, M.D.; and John B. Cummings, Esq.

That year, Charlton Memorial Hospital underwent a corporate reorganization that spawned a parent organization, Charlton

Health System, Inc., and Prospect Properties, Inc., established to conduct real-estate and business activities in support of Charlton Memorial Hospital, Inc. The rejuvenated hospital "cell" had split twice in response to external stimuli and was on its way to creating a complex new organism.

This was the Reagan era, and the mantra was free enterprise and deregulation. Paradoxically, hospitals had to make their way in this brave new world while still tethered by lilliputian rules and regulations. Dreyer described the ambivalent situation by quoting futurist John Naisbitt, who had written, "We are living in the time of the parenthesis, a time between eras." To which Dreyer added:

For 1984 and the years beyond, plans and programs will be developed which are in step with that marketplace setting of today. In- and outpatient services of all kinds, offsetting expensive inpatient services wherever possible, birthing center services, and other such progressive programs must be developed as soon as possible. Dr. Arthur Anctil believes Dreyer sought to stay "one step ahead of those [external influences] who were trying to seize the reins." It was the surest path to maintaining Charlton's independence. "That's why he worked so hard at incorporating physicians into management and onto

Auxiliary leaders: Carol O'Connell, Pauline Duquette; Jean Bogan; Sheila Salvo; with Marge Kenney; and Carol Schwartz

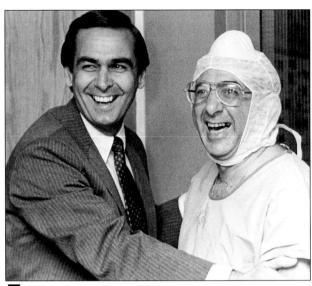

Fall River Mayor Carlton Viveiros and James Sabra, MD share a laugh

Also, two new positions were created at the hospital. Elaine Anderson, R.N., director of nursing, was promoted to Charlton's executive vice president, freeing Dreyer to devote more time and attention to overall system operations, strategic planning, and community and regional affairs. Anderson assumed responsibility for daily operations of the 383-bed hospital, which employed 1,500 people with an annual budget of $57 million. Sydney Rosen, M.D., a thirty-three-year veteran of Charlton, was named medical director, responsible for overall management of the medical staff, quality assessment, and medical-education programs.

In August 1985 the historic Borden Building was spared demolition by Borden Associates, a partnership between Charlton Health System, Inc., and Hanover Associates and earmarked for a $1 million renovation. The first floor would continue to serve as the SurgiCenter, while the upper four floors would be converted into leased offices for an estimated twenty physicians. Erected in 1908, the Borden Building was Union Hospital's flagship and a tangible reminder of Charlton's rich heritage.

the board of trustees," Anctil said. "The idea was, 'Let's manage together.'" In short, it was better to hang together than to hang separately.

That philosophy was carried beyond Fall River in 1985 when Charlton Health System joined with hospitals in nearby communities to form the Southeastern Massachusetts Alliance of Hospitals (later the Gateway Alliance). The goal of the alliance, composed of Morton Hospital (Taunton), Brockton and South Shore hospitals (Weymouth), Tobey (Wareham), and Saint Luke's Hospital (Middleboro), was to "study and promote cost-effective ways to provide quality health care, including educating the public in the effective use of health-care services." CHS also joined the Yankee Alliance, a group of eleven New England hospitals, and continued attempts to forge new alliances with Saint Anne's in Fall River and Saint Luke's in New Bedford.

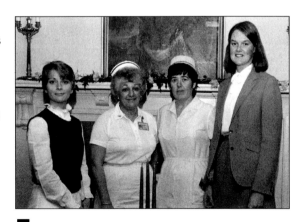

Diane Silvia, RN; Delores Furtado, LPN; Justine Lima, LPN; and Elaine Anderson, RN, executive VP and COO, celebrate LPN week in the Mooney Auditorium of the Elizabeth House.

# Technology and Innovative Programs

$\mathcal{B}$ells and whistles notwithstanding, the raison d'etre of Charlton Memorial Hospital and its permutations was to serve the greater Fall River population, which now tended to be older and prone to degenerative diseases. Increased longevity brought with it not just the gift of life but a greater demand for cardiac, cancer, and

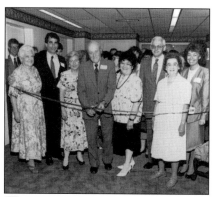

Elsie Frank, U.S. Congressman Barney Frank's mother; Alan Solomont; Mrs. Carrington Lloyd; Clem Dowling; Rita Wood; Frederic C. Dreyer, Jr.; Ethel O'Brien; and Marcia Liggin at the dedication of the Charlton Skilled Nursing Facility, 1989.

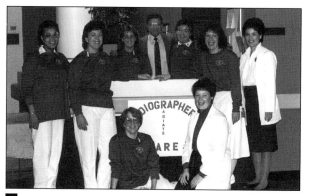

Jack Shah, MD and his staff in radiology, 1985

rehabilitative services. It called for more outreach capability for the homebound and poor. And it signaled a need for preventive medicine to push back the onset of illness.

From 1983 on, several programs were introduced that addressed not only Fall River's senior population but citizens of all ages. That year the Level II nursery debuted to service infants needing close observation and treatment— infants, for example, born prematurely or with drug dependency. It was one of only eight in the state equipped with the latest diagnostic and therapeutic

services. It featured specially trained staff and a neonatologist. Later it became the only such unit in the state to supply a complete range of services.

Charlton's cancer-management program was enhanced in 1985 when the new oncology unit opened at Brayton 3 North. The unit staff employed a team approach in caring for the physical, psycho-social, and emotional needs of patients and their families. The specially trained nurses received ongoing education through Charlton's affiliation with the Dana-Farber Cancer Institute in Boston. Patient rooms were painted in reassuring soft blues, pinks, and mauves, while the curtains were decorated with trees and billowy clouds.

Early in 1986, the emergency department introduced Charlton Plus, an "express care service for

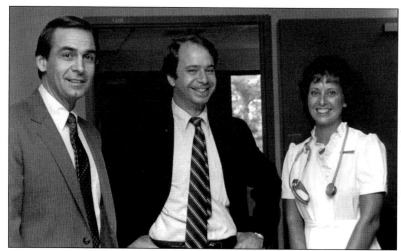

Carlton Viveiros, mayor of the City of Fall River, tours the emergency department with Steven Turbiner, MD and Colette Sirois, RN

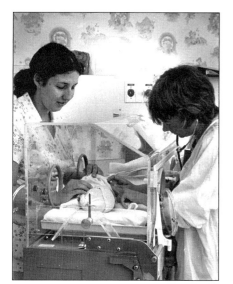

■ *Linda Morais, RN, and Donna Jean Walker, MD, work in the Level II Nursery.*

patients with minor health problems." Charlton Plus was staffed by physicians and nurses from the emergency department, and it was open from 9:00 a.m. to 9:00 p.m. seven days a week. It included five private examining rooms and a waiting area decorated in pastel colors. Major credit cards were accepted, and a discount was offered to patients paying cash. "McMedic" found an instant niche.

The following year, Charlton ventured into a new arena when it introduced Work Med

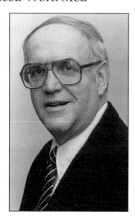

■ *Arthur Marchand, Jr., chairman, Charlton Memorial Hospital Foundation, 1987-1988*

Occupational Health Service, an outgrowth of Charlton's own in-house efforts to reduce worker compensation costs. Work Med helped businesses treat and rehabilitate their injured workers, educate their employees about job safety, and institute policies and procedures complying with federal and state occupational health laws. Charlton Work Med clients now number more than four hundred.

Historically, one of Charlton's chief assets has been its diagnostic services, which range from radiology imaging to cardiac catherization. Diagnostics are done on site or through Charlton Diagnostics, a full-service outpatient laboratory next to the hospital. Cardiac catherization, introduced in 1991, anchors other tests and provides precise data regarding heart or vascular disease. Charlton is one of a handful of community hospitals to offer the procedure.

A recent development, according to Dr. Anctil, is joint-replacement therapy. "It's a big thing," he said. "The community is aging, and there's a

lot of degenerative joint disease. Charlton has some young orthopedic surgeons who are very, very good." For most people, Anctil added, Charlton virtually has become one-stop shopping. "People don't have to leave home. They can get just about anything they need right here."

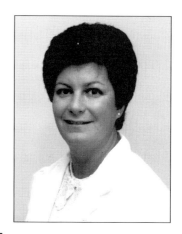

■ *Liz Griffin, director, laboratory*

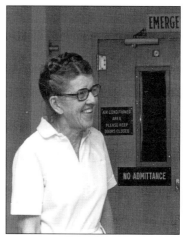

■ *Eunice McDonald, RN, manager emergency department*

# A Matter of Pride

*D*uring the 1980s, Charlton kept its employees and other readers informed about the latest topics of interest in the medical world largely through the *Pride* newsletter. In 1984 neonatologist Donna Jean Walker launched an attack on smoking in pregnancy, pointing out that cigarette smoke contained up to 4,000 chemicals and could reduce the oxygen content in the fetal blood by nearly 20 percent. Many of the chemicals, she added, were carcinogenic. A later article by Charlton nurses probed smoking in adolescence.

In another issue that year, CMH executive vice president Elaine Anderson discussed the potential impact of the new diagnosis-related groups (DRGs), in which a standard rate of payment is set for a Medicare-related service before it is rendered. Hospitals, she said, must find more cost-efficient ways to provide care under DRGs. In 1986 medical malpractice returned to the front burner when an article noted that the state legislature had introduced a bill to cap "pain and suffering" awards at $500,000 while removing limits for "economic" damages. In a 1987 article, Mim Attar, R.N., addressed women on the subject of avoiding the crippling effects of osteoporosis.

Meanwhile, the alphabet-soup world of DRGs, HMOs, PPOs, and PROs continued to act as a catalyst in forcing hospitals to be more market savvy and diversified. Charlton responded quickly with innovations such as Work Med Occupational Health Service and, later, Travel Health, which provided immunizations and counsel for those going out of the country. In addition Charlton and

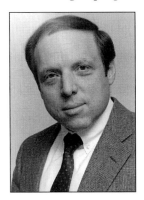

■ *Irwin A. Shaw, Esq., chairman, Charlton Memorial Hospital, 1987-April 1988*

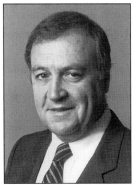

■ *John R. Correiro, chairman, Charlton Memorial Hospital, April 1988-December 1988*

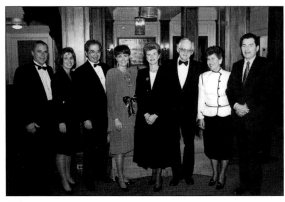

■ *Dr. and Mrs. Vincent F. Geremia, trustee and chief of anesthesiology; Dr. and Mrs. Arthur O. Anctil, trustee and past president of medical staff; Mr. and Mrs. Frederic C. Dreyer, Jr., CHS and CMH president and trustee; and Dr. and Mrs. David S. Greer, dean of Brown Medical School and hospital trustee*

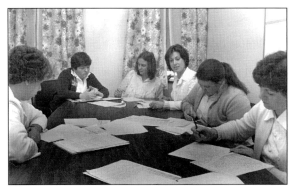

■ *Dianne Peckham, RN; Mary Ann Rooney, RN; Carol Lehoulier; Manuella Medeiros, RN; Margaret Moynagh, RN; and Sue Blackburn, RN*

other hospitals began to share knowledge through regional alliances. The days of individual fiefdoms were over. As Dreyer put it:

There is no longer a question of whether we should enter into prepaid arrangements for health-care services with business and industry, or whether we should network with other hospitals and other providers. The question is with whom, how, and when.

Just how that would have sat with Charles M. Moran is subject to speculation. Moran, the influential, powerful, and intensely loyal former president of the Union board of trustees, died in 1984 at the age of seventy-eight. In his time, the "good doctor" had prevailed. Lawsuits were nonexistent in Massachusetts, and charity loomed large in the medical equation. Community hospitals existed primarily for the local populace, and confidences were rarely traded with a competitor. Some observers gaze back wistfully on those days and note trade-offs have been made over the years. Yet many concede the trade-offs were necessary.

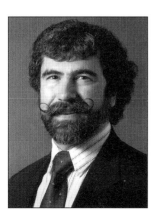

*Stephen S. Kasparian, medical staff president, 1991-1996*

# New Technology for New Times

$\mathcal{S}$ome of those trade-offs involved sophisticated new technology, which was costly and viewed with suspicion by critics. But often critics were won over by the superior results it achieved. In 1984 Charlton purchased a high-powered CO2 laser and an Argon laser for its ambulatory SurgiCenter. They were the first of their kind in the greater Fall River area and a source of great curiosity to those unfamiliar with their operation. Subsequently, it was

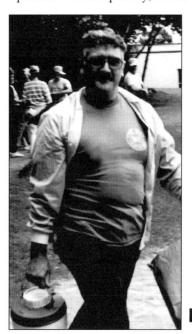

*Joseph Primo, operating room technician, ready for an employee outing*

shown that laser "knives" vaporized dead tissue while cauterizing blood vessels as they cut. With them doctors could complete in twenty minutes what it took hours to do using conventional procedures. Their efficacy was established immediately.

In diagnostic procedures, Charlton's radiology staff demonstrated particular ingenuity in marrying two types of radiological equipment from the old Union and Truesdale sites. When they finished, bi-plane angiographic studies could be performed, which meant frontal and side views of the brain could be mapped simultaneously. This saved time and money for all concerned. In 1978 Charlton took a major step by installing its first CAT body scanner. When it

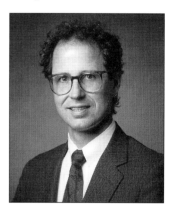

*Frederick W. Schnure, MD, medical staff president, 1989-1990*

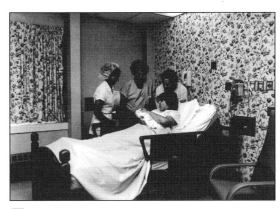

Sharon Bigelow, RN, and Arthur Anctil, MD, with new parents in labor and delivery

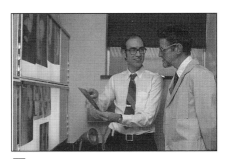

Dr. Kermit Dewey (left) with Arthur Hannifan, senior technician, radiology department, Union-Truesdale Hospital

replaced the scanner six years later, it became only the second hospital in the country to feature the Siemens Somatom DR-2 Body Scanner, a state-of-the-art machine from Germany.

Dr. Anctil, who left a career as a navy doctor to join Union Hospital in 1966, has seen Charlton medical technology explode. "It's mind-boggling," he says. "We started laparoscopic procedures back in 1972, but it was nowhere near as sophisticated as it is today." Today a laparoscopic surgeon views a television monitor while externally manipulating tiny surgical instruments inserted into the body. The laparoscope functions as a mini camera, projecting a magnified image of the patient's internal organs on-screen. Superior hand-eye coordination is critical.

By 1993 Charlton was using laparoscopic surgery for gall-bladder removals, appendectomies, hernia repairs, and hysterectomies. That was only the beginning. The procedure can be adapted to a myriad of conditions.

With laparoscopic surgery, there is less pain, less scar tissue, and shorter hospital stays. Not surprisingly, laparoscopic diagnostics have long been a staple at Charlton.

Another Charlton innovation is central fetal monitoring, which most hospitals do not offer. Monitoring is carried out not only at each of the labor-delivery areas but at the central nursing station. It gives medical personnel more control over "events." Charlton also is equipped with intracranial pressure (ICP) monitors, which are fiber-optic probes inserted into the skull to measure brain swelling. This method is far more accurate and quicker than depending on vital signs. It enables Fall River patients suffering from tumors, hemorrhages, strokes, and head trauma to be treated at Charlton rather than having to be transferred to other facilities.

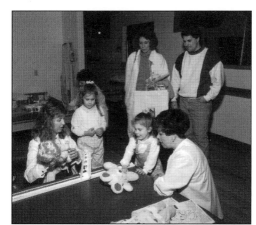

1993 Charlton Memorial Hospital Health Fair "Teddy Bear Clinic": Jay Fontaine, RN; Nicole Peckham; Alyssa Peckham; Diane Peckham, RN; Dot Peckham; Doug Peckham.

# Nursing Comes of Age

*B*y the 1980s, nursing at Charlton was in the middle of a transition period. In the 1970s, it had begun moving from the traditional concept in which nurses filled a subordinate caretaking role to one in which they assumed a degree of autonomy and managerial authority. The new concept was called primary nursing, and it required one-on-one association with an assigned patient from admittance to discharge. Although associate nurses also provided care, the primary nurse was ultimately responsible for the patient's progress and well-being. Dreyer explains:

Members of administration—Elaine Anderson and Nancy Dineen—brought Marie Manthey, author and nurse practitioner and developer of

the practice of primary nursing as it would be practiced in numerous hospitals nationwide, to Charlton on several occasions. Primary nursing promoted high standards of clinical skills, professionalism, and accountability.

The practice led to more advanced initiatives in primary nursing's evolution. The role of the primary practice practitioner or nurse extenders [technical assistants] to experienced registered nurses became much like that of a physician's aid to a physician.

Mary Ann Wordell, a graduate of the Truesdale School of Nursing, remembers the abrupt change in climate when she moved from the more traditional nursing

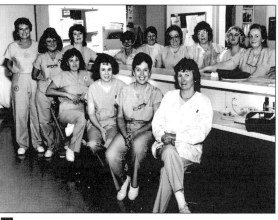

Front row: Judie Lagner, Anne Botelho, Michelle Baker, Debbie Gauthier, Ginny Owen, Gloria Pasqual. Back row: Phyllis Correia, Nancy Wright, Lois Soares, Jan Rousseau, Jackie Levesque, Carolyn Spaulding, Marlene Brabant, 1990

ambiance at Truesdale Hospital to Charlton after the site merger. "The pace was much slower and more hands-on at Truesdale," Wordell said. "Doctors saw patients every day. Union was much bigger, of course, and had a bigger patient load."

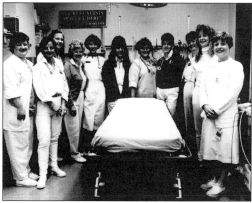

Registered Nurses Jean Mello, Vivian DePerrio, Karen Davis, Gerry Francoeur, Robbie Goff, Pam Carro, Del Nelson, Dianne Raiche, Gail Enos, Robin Liggin, Chris Paquette, 1990

Sundae Rounds during Nurses' Week, May 1995, Erin O'Brien, Lois Spirlet, Cindy Anderson, and Donna Texeira

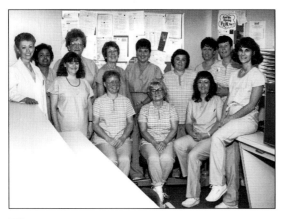

OBS nursing staff. Front row: Registered Nurses Marge Bockman, Kathy Chatterton, Joan Galvin, Judie Farnsworth, Donna Corbean, Karen Leeming. Back row: Fran Logan, RN; Ada White, LPN; Doris Lubold, unit coordinator; Judy McCann, RN; Sandy Mathieu, RN; Tillie Alves, NA; Nancy Cronan, RN, 1990

Wordell moved from head nurse at Truesdale to manager at Charlton. "I didn't get involved a great deal with hands-on care-giving," she recalls. "I became involved with budgets, goal planning, and audits. There were other changes, too, positive things like policy making and professional growth." Where nurses once were expected to nurture patient dependence, they now were exhorted to generate self-reliance in their charges. They were ordered to develop individual plans for patients that included educating them about their illnesses and how to manage them. "This is extremely important with the implementation of DRGs," counseled one *Pride* article. Getting patients "up and out" in the age of prepayments was a top priority. Primary nurses were becoming, in effect, case managers.

# Filling in the Gaps

On a brisk October day in 1992, the Ruth Charlton Mitchell Therapies Center opened in a renovated Catholic gymnasium (previous Sacred Heart Academy) on the Charlton campus. The spacious structure was dedicated to Ruth Charlton Mitchell Masson, whose family had provided financial support to Charlton and its progenitors for seventy years. The original feel of the facility was retained in the original basketball flooring and high ceilings. The center was ideally suited for the task at hand—employing a team approach to rehabilitation. It had plenty of open floor space in which to house departments of physical therapy, occupational therapy, and communication disorders. There also was a second-level exercise track for cardiac-rehabilitation patients.

The Charlton family, represented by Earle P. "Chuck" Charlton, II, had provided a four-year matching grant toward the

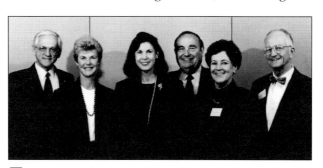

Frederic C. Dreyer, Jr.; Karen Dreyer; Frances Charlton; Earle P. Charlton, II; Grace Lincoln; and Henry Lincoln, MD at the dedication of the Virginia C. Lincoln Center for Women, 1991

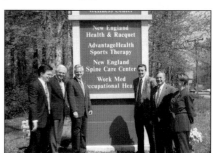

Dedication of the Faunce Corner Wellness Center, 1994

center with the understanding that the Charlton Memorial Hospital Foundation would raise an equal amount through community donations. An additional contribution by Mrs. Masson provided a glassed-in atrium entrance, an idea suggested by "Chuck" Charlton. The center found an immediate constituency and has since become a vital part of the health-care scene in greater Fall River. In a way, it plays counterpoint to the Virginia C. Lincoln Center for Women, an obstetrics department opened at Charlton in 1991 and dedicated to Mrs. Masson's younger sister.

The following year, Charlton oversaw the birth of two more progeny—the Sarah S. Brayton Nursing Care Center and the Charlton Mobile Health Services. The for-profit nursing-care center helped to alleviate a dearth of long-term care facilities in the area by providing short- and long-term rehabilitative care for patients who needed a place to recover beyond the hospital setting. The mobile health services, a forty-foot-long, self-contained van, reached population segments that would not normally have received health care. It furnished free screening and

diagnostic tests plus immunizations and educational services to the elder, indigent, and adolescent populations.

In 1994 the Charlton Wellness Center, a preventive health-care facility, opened in the renovated Faunce Corner Health-Racquet Club in North Dartmouth, Massachusetts. Rehabilitation and medical services were offered along with fitness programs. The new center established a comprehensive sports-medicine program with an eye to serving area high schools and colleges. In addition, the center offered corporate wellness programs to businesses in conjunction with Healthtrax, operator of the center's fitness facility.

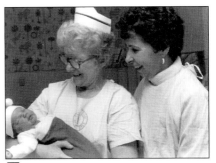

*Eleanor Fanning, LPN and volunteer Lee Huard dress a newborn in Christmas attire.*

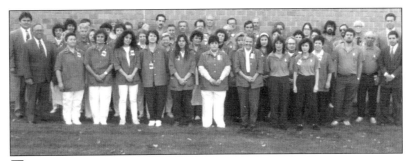

*Environmental services "Gold Award Celebration," 1994*

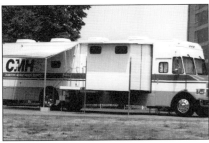

*CMHS's mobile health service van transports education, modern examination and treatment rooms to the community.*

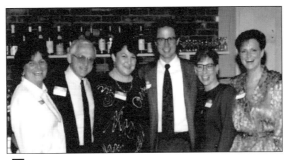

*Nancy Dineen, vice president nursing; Frederic C. Dreyer, Jr.; Rosanne Berwald, MD; Rick Schnure, MD, past president of the medical staff; Joan Roover, vice president and assistant to the president; and Dorothy Allen, vice president of development and marketing early 1990s*

## Charlton Updates Philanthropy

As Charlton Health System evolved into a sprawling regional system, philanthropy became the strict province of professionals—first under the Charlton Health System, now under Southcoast's Center for Philanthropy and Volunteer Service, headed by Vice President Dorothy A. Allen, a certified fund-raising executive (CFRE). Allen says the gift-volunteer time and talent is encouraged as much as financial support. To that end, the center reaches out to the community through written communications, events, open

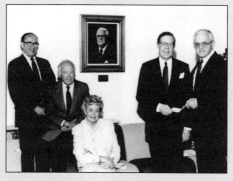

John Dator, Charlton Memorial trustee; Sanford Udis, MD, chief of radiology of Truesdale Clinic; and Betty Welch, business manager of Truesdale Clinic, look on as Paul Dunn, MD presents Frederic C. Dreyer, Jr., CEO of Charlton Health System a donation by the Bud Pierce Foundation.

houses, and the like, to get people involved and informed. It does not wait for contributors, it cultivates them.

"We rely on building relationships that provide sustaining support—for life," Allen says. "We give donors a way to express their commitment to this hospital and this community. The hospital gets needed funds, and the donor gets an opportunity to really make a difference." Some gifts even offer the donor a special dividend: income. As an example, she told of a woman who swapped her low-return stock for a separate higher-earning lifetime annuity. The hospital was able to profitably sell the stock while the woman enhanced her income. "We educate people on their options," Allen says. "Many of the larger gifts are made by people who are seeking tax relief through charitable giving; however, it is in the donor's interest in this organization that really generates the gift."

Another option, an endowed-name fund, allows families to establish a hospital endowment in the family name. Individual family members can make gifts to the fund whenever they choose. The fund is invested by the hospital, and the income can be designated annually for a specific purpose such as cancer, women's health, etc. Allen says the Center for Philanthropy and Volunteer Service currently counts about three thousand living contributors a year, a number that grows annually as more people designate the hospital as a conduit for their community support. Allen says, "It is a most exciting experience to see people give extraordinary levels of their time, talent, and treasure—to hear them say, 'This is my hospital,' makes our mission come alive. "

# The Beat Goes On

By 1994, Charlton Memorial Hospital had become a sprawling complex. It boasted 1,700 employees, more than 200 doctors and an annual budget of $120 million. It had thrived despite the turbulent aftermath of the Union-Truesdale merger and a reduction in the work force attributable to legislative budget constraints and changing medical trends. Yet in the midst of phenomenal growth, Charlton retained its special aura as the "hometown hospital." Fall River families, to whom Charlton had given succor for generations, continued to regard it as an integral part of their lives.

Rick Dreyer could be forgiven if he took Charlton's success a bit personally. As its chief administrator for nearly thirty years, he had shepherded the hospital into the modern age. In terms of drive and dedication, he had few equals. And he did not exclude himself from his commitment to change. In December he handed the reins of the hospital presidency over to Dr. Ronald B. Goodspeed, a forty-eight-year-old internist and pharmacist who had been executive vice president and chief operating officer of Charlton since 1991. The transfer would take effect on January 1, 1995.

Goodspeed, like Dreyer, had a varied and somewhat untraditional background. He had

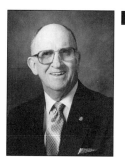
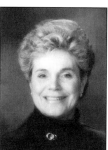
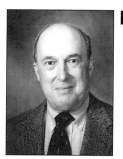
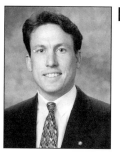
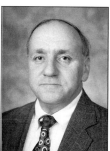

experience in private practice, full-time academic medicine at the University of Connecticut School of Medicine, managed care and administrative medicine. Before coming to Charlton, he worked as assistant vice president and medical director at a health-insurance company, which yielded valuable insights into health care-trends. In his new job, Goodspeed's mission was to provide hospital "leadership and vision" as well as a link to the community. Dreyer, meanwhile, would devote all of his time to Charlton Health System—the parent corporation—as its president and chief executive officer.

As Dreyer and Goodspeed assumed their respective duties, another development was proceeding apace. Regionalization, which Dreyer had pushed for years, was coming to term. The first faint heartbeats had been heard a decade before when the Southeast Massachusetts Alliance of Hospitals and Gateway Alliance were conceived. During the gestation period that followed, Charlton,

Saint Anne's, Saint Luke's (New Bedford), and Tobey (Wareham) hospitals engaged in wide-ranging discussions and limited collaborations.

In 1991, for example, Charlton and Saint Luke's teamed up to serve maternal and neonatal patients. Charlton provided Level II and special care nurseries, while Saint Luke's offered Level 1B and continuing-care nurseries. The hospitals also discussed establishing a regional advanced-life-support service. A year later, a Charlton administration team brainstormed ideas for projects with Saint Luke's. Suggestions included, among others, a joint MRI facility, a joint program in occupational health, and a coordinated psychiatric program headed by Saint Luke's.

In an ensuing letter to Saint Luke's president John Day, Dreyer suggested adoption of "two or more" of the ideas, which could serve as "pilot regionalization initiatives." He further suggested augmenting the CMH-SLH joint study group with additional trustees from both hospitals. "I have spoken with Charlton Health System Board Chairman John Dator and [CMH] hospital Board Chairman Bill Torpey," Dreyer wrote. "Both have agreed it would be advisable to do that." During the same period, Dreyer also recommended hitching regionalization to the Southeast Massachusetts Partnership, a united effort by Fall River, Taunton, New Bedford, and Attleboro mayors and others to develop a strategic economic-development plan for the area.

As time passed, the process of regionalization took on a life of its own. Pressured by a changing economy, hospital privatization, aggressive health plans, and shrinking federal entitlements, Charlton and its allies cleared the obstacles out of the way with dispatch. Finally, on June 9, 1996, the dream became a reality. Everything was in order that summer morning when representatives from Charlton Health System, Saint Luke's Health Care System, and Tobey Health Systems sat down and signed documents creating the Southcoast Health System.

The new entity boasted 3,633 employees and a net patient-service revenue of $287 million. John Day, former Saint Luke's president, became president of Southcoast Health System, while Goodspeed became executive vice president. Dr. Goodspeed also assumed the presidency of Southcoast Hospitals Group. Initial Southcoast plans reflected the recent past as well as the future—some administrative departments would be merged and some jobs consolidated. In addition, Southcoast now eyed an advanced-coronary-care unit where patients could receive sophisticated treatment without leaving "home." Once again, Charlton had reinvented itself and seized the future. President and Emeritus Rick Dreyer foresees even greater changes with "mega-mergers, regional expansions and international systems." Yet the Charlton "mission of caring and serving others will be perpetuated." John Flint would have been pleased. ∎

# *Chronology*

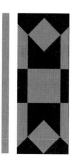

# Charlton Chronology

**1885**  Fall River Hospital is founded on Prospect Street.

**1900**  Union Hospital is born of a merger between Fall River Hospital and the Emergency Hospital. It is located on Prospect and Hanover streets.

**1905**  Dr. Philemon Truesdale purchases Sacred Heart Rectory on the corner of Winter and Pine streets and opens a private hospital.

**1906** Perry Charlton, son of Fall River entrepreneur Earle P. Charlton, is treated for a ruptured appendix and peritonitis at Dr. Truesdale's hospital. He recovers, setting the stage for later philanthropy by the Charlton family.

**1909** Truesdale builds Highland Hospital, a neocolonial structure with verandas, at the end of Highland Avenue.

**1911** Union Hospital becomes one of the first hospitals in New England to establish outpatient and social-services departments.

**1912** Union Hospital joins in establishing a district nursing association, primarily to combat high infant mortality in the Fall River area.

Union introduces the "well baby" clinic and sets up stations throughout the city to dispense pasteurized milk.

The Truesdale Nursing School is established by Dr. Ralph French.

Hicks House (nursing quarters) is built with funds provided by grateful former patient Maria Hicks.

**1914** Dr. Matthew Tennis, Union Hospital's first full-time "roentgenologist" assumes duties.

The Truesdale Clinic is established on Rock Street. It is inspired by the Mayo Clinic concept of group practice.

**1915** Highland Hospital goes public and is renamed Truesdale Hospital.

**1917** Union Hospital completes construction of the Stevens Clinic, named after benefactor Elizabeth Stevens.

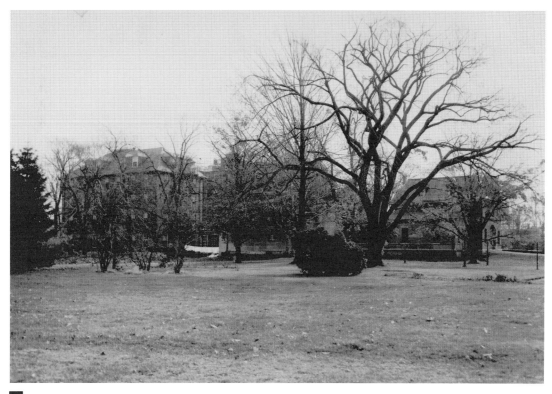

An early photograph of the Brayton estate where
Union Hospital would be built

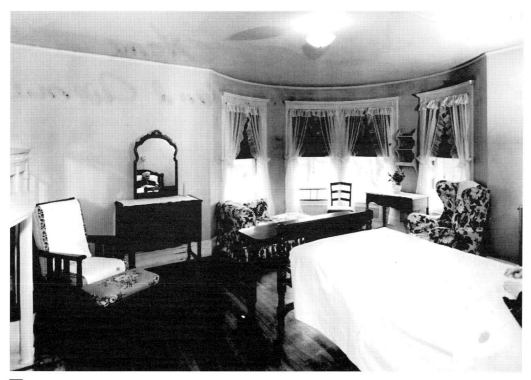

A patient room at the Truesdale Convalescent Home which was formerly
Dr. Truesdale's home

**1918** During worldwide epidemic of influenza, Union Hospital sets aside an isolation ward to receive the stricken.

**1922** An electrocardiograph is added to Union Hospital's outpatient department. Cardiologist Clifton B. Leech joins the medical staff.

**1923** A south wing is added to Truesdale Hospital, thanks to benefactors Earle P. Charlton and Eva McGowen.

**1927** A surgical wing is completed at Truesdale. Earle P. Charlton financed the entire project.

The Goff Memorial Ward is completed at Union Hospital. It is funded by Elizabeth Stevens.

**1929** The Grush property west of Union Hospital is purchased.

**1931** Mitchell House (nursing quarters) opens at Truesdale.

**1933** Elizabeth House, a nursing residence with classrooms, opens. It is funded by the late Elizabeth Stevens.

**1935** Union Hospital initiates an experimental group-hospital plan in an effort to lower medical costs.

The Union Hospital Home for Invalids opens. Buildings, property, and renovations are the gift of Mr. and Mrs. Rudolf F. Haffenreffer.

Dr. Truesdale performs "upside-down" stomach operation.

A fourth floor is added to Truesdale Hospital.

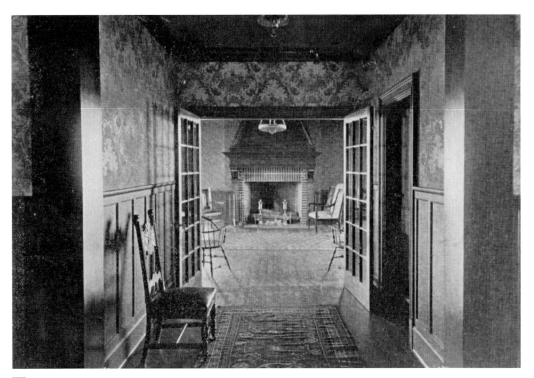

Interior of the Mitchell House

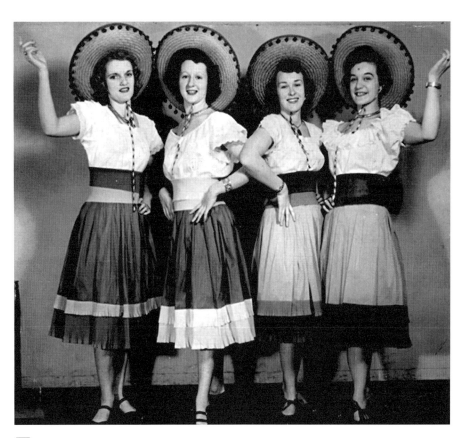

Bernice Brown, Barbara Mersier, Ethel Wescott and Colette Arkison in the 1950 Union Hospital Follies

**1938**  Union Hospital provides shelter and care during the New England hurricane of 1938.

**1943**  Truesdale Hospital becomes one of nine Massachusetts hospitals designated as a major blood collector for the war effort.

**1948**  Union Hospital's Dr. Leonard Bolen develops a method of diagnosing cancer through the blood.

**1949**  Ruth Mitchell, Earle P. Charlton's daughter, donates the family library of their Westport Harbor home to Truesdale Hospital.

Union Hospital's annual report suggests the possibility of consolidation with Truesdale Hospital.

**1950**  Statistics reveal the infant mortality rate in Fall River has dropped from 202 deaths per 1,000 births in 1915 to 23 deaths, largely as a result of untiring efforts by Union Hospital and the District Nursing Association.

**1955**  Union Hospital board of trustees president John S. Brayton donates to the hospital—with siblings Flint, Anthony, and Edith—the six-and-a-half-acre Brayton estate at Highland Avenue and New Boston Road.

The Jacob Ziskind Laboratory opens at Union Hospital, thanks to funding by the estate of Jacob Ziskind, whose brother, Abraham, was a former trustee.

**1956**  The Union-Truesdale Hospital Building Fund raises $1,350,000.

Truesdale Hospital opens an isotope laboratory.

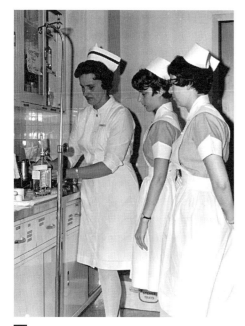

■ *Lorraine Davol, RN, MS, prepares IV medications with student nurses at Union Hospital.*

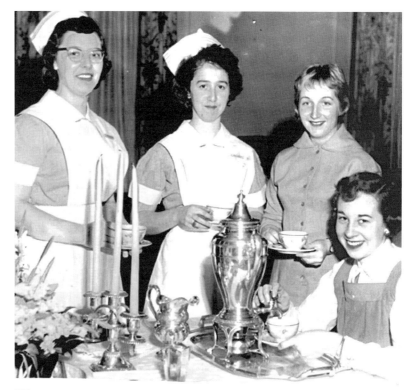

■ *Truesdale nurses' alumnae tea at the Mitchell House attended by Janet Kaszynski Pereira, Ann Hanley Crane, Joan Wolowiec Lynch and Elizabeth O'Rourke Lee, circa 1956*

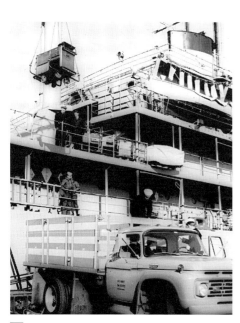

■ *A donation of medical equipment to an underdeveloped country transported by the navy*

**1957**    A community survey by Union-Truesdale administrators recommends the merger of the hospitals into one entity with 350 beds.

**1958**    The National Nursing Accreditation Service grants the Union School of Nursing accreditation.

**1959**    Union Hospital's sixty-bed Brayton Building is completed.

Truesdale Hospital adds an east wing.

**1961**    Union Hospital installs a television fluoroscope, perhaps the third such diagnostic tool in the United States.

Union Hospital purchases property from Prospect Street south to Maple Street.

**1962**    The south wing of Union Hospital's Brayton Building is completed.

Hospital consultant Anthony J.J. Rourke, M.D., recommends Union and Truesdale hospitals consolidate but retain their individual sites.

**1963**    Union Hospital establishes the Department of Medical Education, a postgraduate program, under Dr. John C. Corrigan.

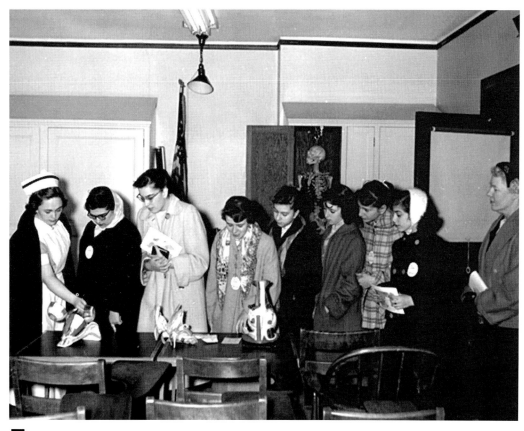

■ *Students are introduced to nursing at Truesdale, circa 1950s*

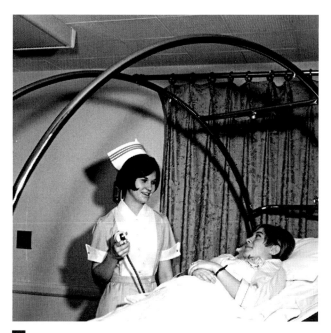

■ *Truesdale Hospital, circa 1960s*

**1966**  Truesdale opens a coronary intensive-care unit with cardiac-monitoring equipment, the first of its kind in the area.

The Jacob Ziskind Lab gets an addition.

**1968**  Union, Truesdale, and Saint Anne's hospitals begin preliminary talks regarding consolidation.

**1970**  Union, Truesdale, and Saint Anne's nursing schools merge, creating the Fall River Diploma School of Nursing.

**1971**  Union Hospital's acute-care Charles Moran Building is completed, along with a state-of-the-art boiler plant.

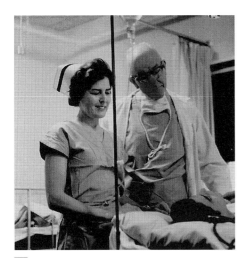

Virginia Zillis, RN, and Daniel Gallery, MD, chief of surgery

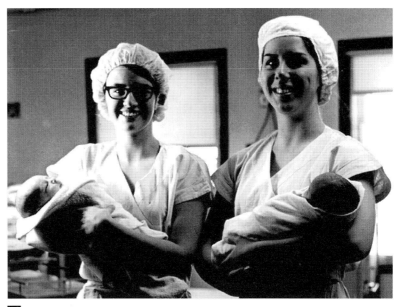

Nurses Nancy Turner and Gail Rinaldi in Truesdale's nursery

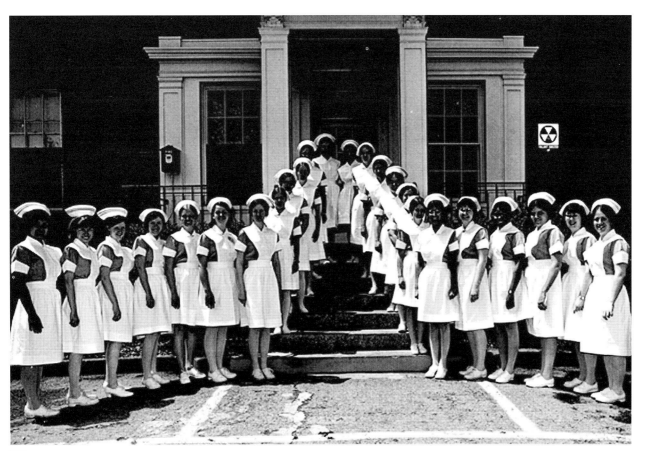

Class of 1972, the last to graduate from Union Hospital School of Nursing

**1972**  Discussions on hospital consolidation deepen to include state and regional officials.

Saint Anne's Hospital backs out of consolidation with Truesdale Hospital.

**1974**  Truesdale merger with Hussey Hospital falls through.

**1975**  Union and Truesdale hospitals consolidate, retaining their individual sites and becoming Union-Truesdale Hospital.

**1978**  A CAT body scanner is installed.

**1979**  The Charlton family donates $1 million to the Charlton Memorial Hospital building fund.

Union-Truesdale Hospital is renamed Charlton Memorial Hospital.

**1980**  The vascular laboratory opens.

Charlton trades pediatric services for obstetrical services with Saint Anne's.

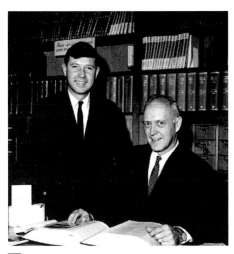

■ *Administrator F. Bliss Winn and Vernon Bradbury, treasurer of Truesdale Hospital*

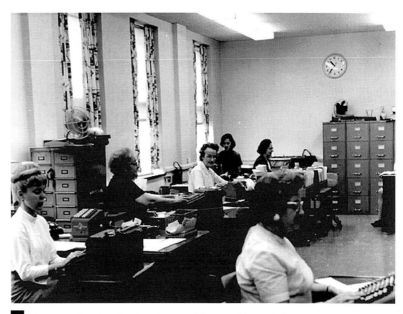

■ *Secretaries in the business office at Truesdale*

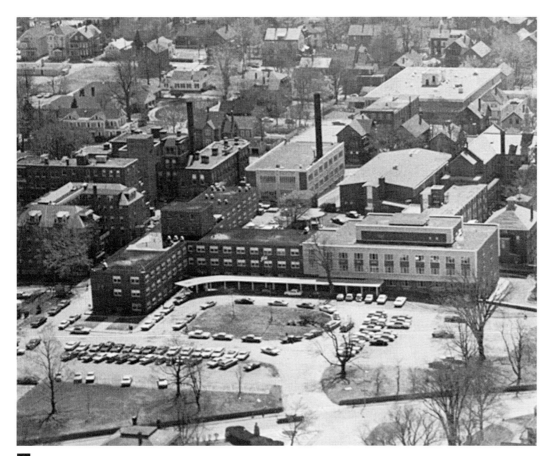

■ *Aerial of Union Hospital, circa early 1970s*

**1983**   Charlton Memorial Hospital merges at one site, with the former Truesdale Hospital being sold to developers.

The Atwood Building, a five-story patient-care facility, is completed.

The Mitchell Building is completed, introducing a "one-stop shopping" concept in maternity care with seven labor-delivery-recovery rooms and a Level II nursery.

**1984**   A comprehensive four-phase cardiac-rehabilitation program is introduced.

Charlton Health System, Inc., is established.

Laser surgery services are offered at SurgiCenter.

**1986**   Charlton Plus, a convenience-care center in the emergency department, is established.

**1987**   Charlton's Occupational Health Service, serving client companies in southeastern Massachusetts, is established.

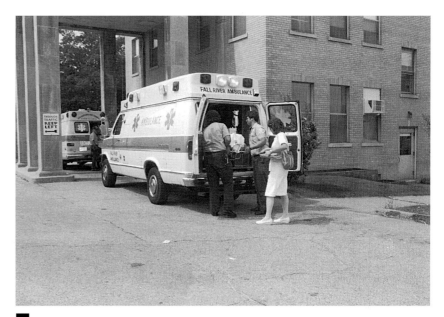

■ *Moving patients from the Truesdale site*

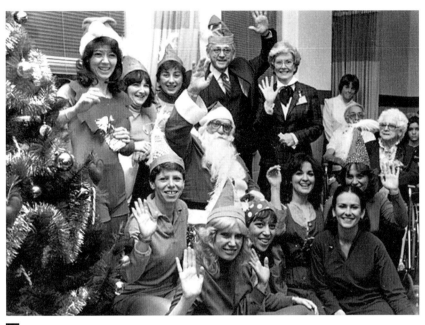

Union-Truesdale Christmas party

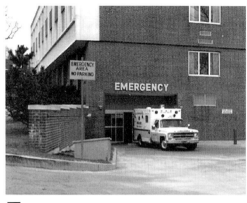

Entrance to the emergency room
before the Atwood Building was added

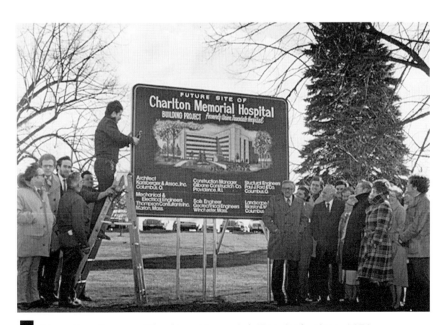

Plans for the new Charlton Memorial Hospital, circa 1979

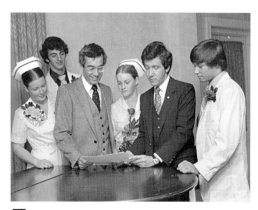

Debra A. Desmarais, Brad Morse, Dr.
Charles Mandell, Robin Hodkinson,
Tom Cinquini and Paul Lemaire

1988    Mobile magnetic-resonance imaging is introduced as part of a regional consortium of eight hospitals in southeastern Massachusetts.

1989    The Skilled Nursing Facility, a forty-five-bed onsite Level II unit, opens.

1990    Southeast Rehabilitation Center, a twenty-bed on-site facility, is opened.

1991    Charlton cardiac catherization unit opens.
        Virginia C. Lincoln Center for Women opens.

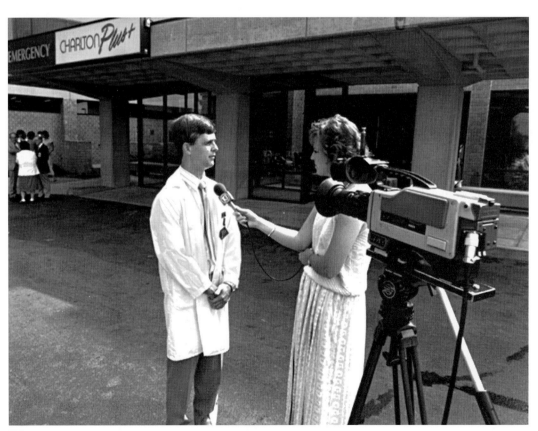

■ *Wayne Christianson, DO, chairman of the emergency medicine department describes the new Charlton Plus program which offered walk-in services for non-emergency patients, circa 1980s.*

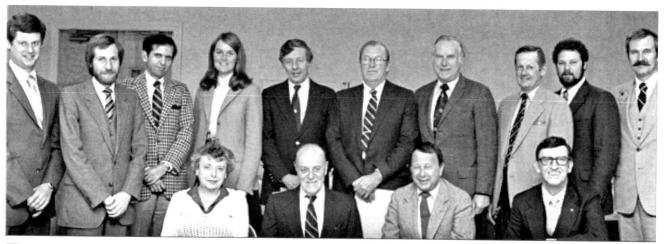

*Charlton Memorial leadership, circa 1980s (sitting): Ruth Hurley, trustee; Clement J. Dowling, trustee and clerk of the corporation; Alex Friedman, MD; William F. Torpey, president; (standing): Edward Dobbs; Arthur J. Sampson, vice president; Harvey Reback, MD; Elaine F. Anderson, senior vice president; Robert F. Laing, trustee; Arthur Smith, MD; Francis T. Meagher, Esq., trustee; Francis James, MD, past president; Richard Kisner, administrative resident; Robert McDonald, vice president*

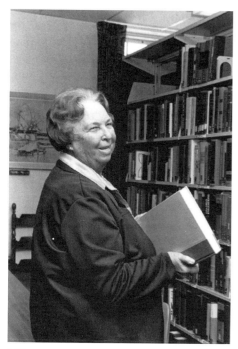

*Ruth B. Merritt, former president of the Woman's Board and trustee of Union Hospital, 1981*

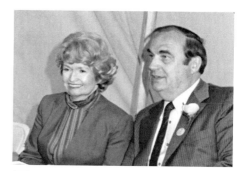

*Margaret Heckler, secretary of HEW, and Earle P. "Chuck" Charlton at the Atwood Building dedication*

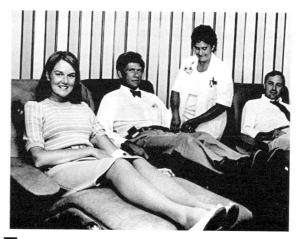

*Elaine F. Anderson, Dr. Jeremy Worthington, Jane Rego and John Gurney in the blood bank*

1992    Ruth Charlton Mitchell Therapies Center opens.

1993    Fixed MRI unit is established.

CMHS's mobile health service van begins.

The Sarah S. Brayton Nursing Care Center opens in north Fall River.

1994    The Charlton Wellness Center is established in North Dartmouth, MA.

1995    Linden Tree Community Medical Services Center established in Portsmouth, RI.

1996    Charlton Health System, Inc. merges with Saint Luke's Health Care System, of New Bedford, MA, and Tobey Health Systems, of Wareham, MA, to form Southcoast Health System.

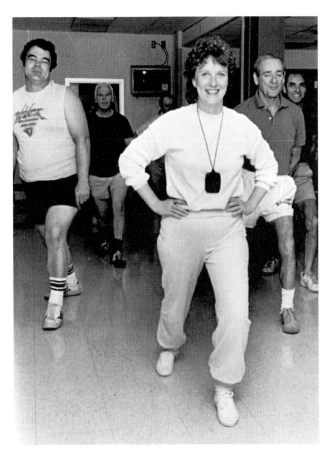

Joyce Grusmark, assistant director of physical
therapy leads an exercise class

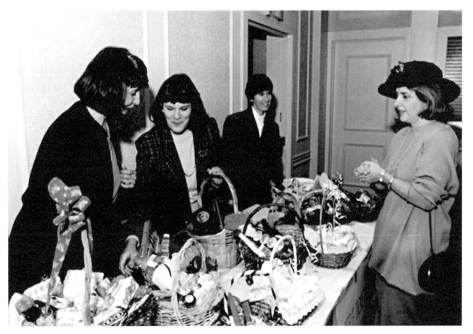

Elizabeth Fitton, Jennifer Vergnani, Madeline O'Brien and Linda Monchik
at the donor luncheon, 1992.

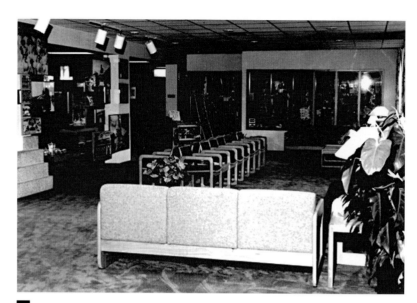

■ Charlton Memorial Hospital lobby, circa 1990s

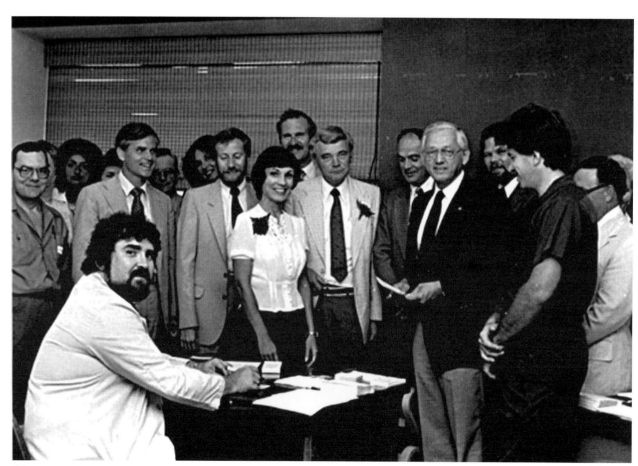

■ Opening of the Charlton Memorial Hospital credit union

# Union Hospital 1900–1975

## Union Board of Trustees

### Presidents

| | |
|---|---|
| John D. Flint | 1900–01, 1904–05 |
| John S. Brayton | 1901–02 |
| Dr. Robert T. Davis | 1902–04 |
| Elias A. Tuttle | 1905–07 |
| Richard P. Borden | 1907–13, 1923–42 |
| W. Frank Shove | 1913–23 |
| John S. Brayton, III | 1942–61 |
| Charles M. Moran | 1961–74 |
| George R. Boyce, Esq. | 1974–75 |

## Recent Union Administrators

| | |
|---|---|
| Jennie Smithies, R.N. | 1942–54 |
| L.V. Ragsdale, M.D. | 1955–66 |
| George M. Jackson | 1966–69 |
| Frederic C. Dreyer, Jr. | 1969–75 |

# Truesdale Hospital 1917-1975

## Truesdale Board of Trustees

### Presidents/Chairmen

| | |
|---|---|
| Ralph W. French, M.D. | 1917–21, 1940–42 |
| Frederick R. Barnes, M.D. | 1922–24 |
| Earle P. Charlton | 1925–29 |
| John H. Lindsey, M.D. | 1930–32 |
| Judge James M. Morton, Jr. | 1933–39 |
| Warren G. Atwood, M.D. | 1943–46 |
| Frederick M. Mitchell | 1947–53 |
| John B. Cummings, Esq. | 1953–65 |
| Philip S. Brayton | 1966–71* |
| Robert P. Truesdale | 1972–75 |

*During Philip S. Brayton's tenure the position was changed from president to chairman.

## Recent Truesdale Administrators

| | |
|---|---|
| Hayden Deaner | 1954–68 |
| F. Bliss Winn | 1968–75 |

## Recent Truesdale Presidents

| | |
|---|---|
| Robert S. Murray | 1970–75 |

# Charlton Health System Inc.

# Charlton Memorial Hospital

(known as Union-Truesdale Hospital 1975–1979)

## Chairmen

| | |
|---|---|
| Joseph A. Faria | 1975–76 |
| George R. Boyce, Esq. | 1976–78 |
| John F. Dator | 1978–80 |
| Donald Ramsbottom | 1980–86 |
| George R. Boyce, Esq. | 1986 |
| Irwin A. Shaw | 1986-88 |
| John R. Correiro | 1988 |
| William J. Torpey | 1988–92 |
| Carol A. O'Connell | 1993–95 |
| William H. Lapointe | 1996 |

## Charlton Health System, Inc. *
## Chairmen

| | |
|---|---|
| Arthur Marchand, Jr. | 1986–88 |
| John F. Dator | 1988–92 |
| Barry Robbins | 1993–95 |
| John M. Almeida | 1996–96 |

*Prior to 1992 the parent corporation, was Charlton Memorial Hospital Foundation.

## Charlton Health System, Inc.

*President and CEO*

| | |
|---|---|
| Frederic C. Dreyer, Jr. | 1986–1996 |

## Presidents of the Medical Staff

| | |
|---|---|
| Thomas J. Muldowney, M.D. | 1975–77 |
| Philip W. Smith, M.D. | 1977–78 |
| Arthur O. Anctil, M.D. | 1978–79 |
| Arthur O. Anctil, M.D. | 1980–81 |
| Francis M. James, M.D. | 1981–82 |
| Lawrence F. Audino, M.D. | 1983–85 |
| Herbert S. Rubin, M.D. | 1985–88 |
| Frederick W. Schnure, M.D. | 1989–90 |
| Stephen S. Kasparian, M.D. | 1991–96 |

# Charlton Memorial Hospital

*President and CEO*

| | |
|---|---|
| Frederic C. Dreyer, Jr. | 1975–94 |
| Ronald B. Goodspeed, M.D. | 1994–96 |

# Auxiliary Presidents

| | |
|---|---|
| Betty Bounakes | 1965–1968 |
| Elsie Wildnauer | 1969–1970 |
| Sheila Salvo | 1971–1973 |
| Dorothy Stafford | 1973–1975 |
| Sue Hutton | 1975–1977 |
| Tish James | 1977–1978 |
| Beverly Udis | 1978–1979 |
| Sheila Salvo | 1979–1980 |
| Jean Bogan | 1980–1981 |
| Carol O'Connell | 1981–1982 |
| Pauline Duquette | 1982–1983 |
| Elizabeth Mercer | 1983–1984 |
| Carolyn Kaiser | 1984–1985 |
| Patricia Bartek | 1985–1986 |
| Marcia Zuehlke | 1986–1987 |
| Edith Samson | 1987–1988 |
| Claire Thompson | 1988–1989 |
| Carole Waxler | 1989–1990 |
| Margaret Geldart | 1990–1991 |
| Claire Thompson | 1991–1992 |
| Patricia Jacques | 1992–1993 |
| Elizabeth Fitton | 1993–1994 |
| Emily Myles | 1994–1996 |
| Ann Petrella | 1996–1997 |

# Charlton Memorial Hospital Foundation
(Charlton Memorial Hospital's subsidiary, CMH Foundation was organized in 1992)
Chairmen

| | |
|---|---|
| Clifford R. Carlson | 1990-1993 |
| William J. Torpey | 1993-1995 |
| Agatha St. Amour | 1995-1996 |

## Hospital Construction
## Union-Charlton

| | |
|---|---|
| 1888 | Fall River Hospital (renovation) |
| 1908 | Main (Borden) Building |
| 1917 | Stevens Clinic |
| 1927 | Goff Memorial (fifth floor, Stevens Building) |
| 1933 | Elizabeth House (nurse's quarters) |
| 1934 | Home for Convalescents (renovation) |
| 1959 | Brayton Building |
| 1962 | South wing, Brayton Building |
| 1971 | Moran Building |
| 1971 | Power plant |
| 1983 | Atwood Building |
| 1983 | Mitchell Building (renovation) |
| 1989 | Skilled Nursing Facility |
| 1990 | Southeast Rehabilitation Center |
| 1991 | Charlton cardiac catherization unit |
| 1991 | Virginia C. Lincoln Center for Women |
| 1992 | Ruth Charlton Mitchell Therapies Center |
| 1993 | Sarah S. Brayton Nursing Care Center |
| 1993 | Fixed MRI unit |
| 1994 | Charlton Wellness Center |
| 1995 | Linden Tree Family Health Center |

## Hospital Construction
## Truesdale

| | |
|---|---|
| 1910 | Highland Hospital |
| 1912 | Hicks House (nurse's quarters) |
| 1915 | Truesdale Clinic |
| 1923 | South wing |
| 1927 | Charlton surgery wing |
| 1931 | Mitchell House (nurse's quarters) |
| 1938 | Fourth floor added |
| 1947 | Ida S. Charlton Medical Library (imported from Westport) |
| 1959 | East wing |

# Sources

Fell, Ernest, M., M.D., "A Short History of the Union Hospital in Fall River" (unpublished manuscript) 1979

Union Hospital *Log* (newsletters)

Charlton Memorial Hospital *Pride* (newsletters)

Union Hospital annual reports

Truesdale Hospital annual reports

Charlton Memorial Hospital annual reports

Silvia, Philip T., *Victorian Vistas: Fall River, 1886–1900*, Smith Printing Company 1988

Silvia, Philip T., *Victorian Vistas: Fall River, 1901–1911*, Smith Printing Company,1992

Fall River Historical Society

Fall River Public Library

The *Fall River Herald News*

Bordley, James, and Harvey, A. Mcgehee, *Two Centuries of American Medicine*, Saunders Company, 1976

Golden, Janet, and Long, Diana, *The American General Hospital*, Cornell University Press 1989

Cassedy, James H., *Medicine in America: A Short History*, Johns Hopkins University Press 1991

Singer, Charles Joseph, and Underwood, Edgar Ashworth, *A Short History of Medicine*, Oxford University Press 1962

Rosenberg, Charles E., *The Care of Strangers: The Rise of the American Hospital System*, Basic Books 1987

*The Best American Essays 1996*, Houghton Mifflin Company 1996

Manchester, William, *The Glory and the Dream*, Little, Brown and Company 1973

*The Timetables of History*, Simon & Schuster, Inc., 1979